LOVING HANNAH

childhood cancer treatment from the other side of the bed

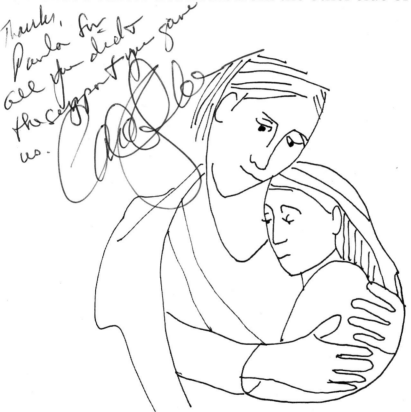

Thanks, Paula for all you did to the support you gave us.

a memoir by
CAROL GLOVER, MSN, FNP-C

Loving Hannah
childhood cancer treatment from the other side of the bed

ISBN: 978-1-936447-70-1

Produced by Maine Authors Publishing, Rockland, Maine

Printed in the United States of America

Cover art: Peggy Murray - Lee, New Hampshire

DEDICATION

This book is dedicated to all of the skilled and knowledgeable nurses of the Pediatric Inpatient Unit and Maine Children's Cancer Program who provided outstanding care for us. And to Molly Schwenn, MD, Craig Hurwitz, MD, Virginia Hamilton, MD, and Annie Rossi, MD, the physicians whose knowledge, skills, and commitment to caring for children and families with cancer is unsurpassed. Thank you.

IN REMEMBRANCE OF

MATT SARNO
ANDREA
DANIEL
ALANA

TABLE OF CONTENTS

FORWARD

October 4, 2002

Today my eleven-year-old daughter, Hannah, completed the last of four rounds of chemotherapy to treat acute myeloid leukemia. It has been 134 days since my world spun off its axis with a phone call. We (me during the week and my husband, Mike, on the weekends) lived with her at the Barbara Bush Children's Hospital at Maine Medical Center in Portland, Maine. For 83 of those days, Hannah was an inpatient in either a positive-pressure room or one of the other rooms on the pediatric unit reserved for children with cancer.

Enduring this trial meant segmenting my life into a series of overlapping but separate functions:

- helping Hannah cope with treatments, transfusions, and medications along with all of their attendant side effects;

- trying to protect her from infections or secondary hospitalization problems that could prove fatal;

- supporting Hannah through all of the emotional effects of treatment, the loneliness of isolation, and just normal "preteenism";

- mourning with her as she struggled with weight loss, hair loss, and innocence loss;

- keeping home and household running while not being at home;

- continuing to be a mom to my fifteen-year-old daughter and wife to my husband while rarely seeing them;

- being a health care professional in a health care setting with a nonprofessional role; and

- finally, fighting daily not to succumb to the constant gut-gnawing pain and fear that this unique person who is my daughter might die.

Although there were many days when I thought the task would be beyond my capabilities, there were also unimagined gifts. Learning to just *live* every day even though I had lost control over many parts of my life was a true gift. Bearing the pain, anger, and grief, which were my daily companions, and realizing that I could still survive, made me stronger. Struggling to match the courage of my deeply spiritual eleven-year-old fighter named Hannah became my life and my reward.

For a parent, facing childhood cancer may be one of the ultimate lessons in living in the here and now. Each moment of every day, once the diagnosis of cancer is made, provides either a challenge to overcome and survive or a respite from those challenges. Being forced to live so completely in each moment gave me a dizzying and profound glimpse into my own innermost being.

As a Nurse Practitioner, my experience of Hannah's cancer treatment was different from that of other parents. I had a different relationship with my fellow health care professionals, and understood many of the risks and problems more completely. It didn't change the fact that I was, through all of this, first and foremost Hannah's mom, but it meant that I had a wider view of the issues involved in her treatment and her care.

Although I always tried, in my professional role, to be sensitive and aware of the needs of patients and their families when they were experiencing illness, I did not understand the feeling of powerlessness and despair that comes with a diagnosis of cancer. My medical knowledge was both an asset and a burden. I knew more than many other parents might know, which helped me to anticipate potential problems, but that knowledge also increased my fear and anxiety about those potential dangers. The most important lesson I learned was that the care of any patient is more about the importance of healing than it is about the treatment process. Although I felt I knew all of these parts of nursing in my practice experience, I had never lived them day after day.

The following story is about my journey through Hannah's illness and treatment, the toll it took on our lives, and the gifts it gave to us. We had to confront issues that we never expected or wanted to face, but through it we gained richer and more meaningful lives. The decision to chronicle the experiences of this journey evolved not only from my need to process the experience through writing, but from a desire to share it with others. I hope it may help another parent facing childhood cancer, and perhaps it might also give health care providers a deeper insight into and a better understanding of the world in which families of children with cancer live.

—Carol Clover, MSN, FNP-C

Chapter 1

ANSWERS

I had been waiting for the test results all morning, but when the phone finally rang, I had to force myself to answer it.

The doctor we saw yesterday asked, "May I speak with Carol Glover?"

"This is she."

"Your daughter has cancer. It is some type of leukemia, but we don't know yet which kind."

The words punched the air out of my lungs; breathing hurt. "Your daughter has cancer." Cancer! I teetered on the edge of an abyss. I grabbed the desk to keep from falling out of my chair. I felt as if I was going to vomit and faint at the same time. In dire situations your life is supposed to flash before your eyes, but all I saw was Hannah's life; every moment since I first held her as a newborn in my arms, was compressed into that second.

Pain, from crushing the phone in my hand, brought me back to the words I was hearing.

"Where do you want to go for treatment?"

I had no clue. Nothing had prepared me to make such a decision. I couldn't think; I could only hear my heart pounding. This wasn't a professional decision. I wasn't deciding the medical plan or outcome. I had no control. I was a mom, and I was being asked to decide where my daughter would be admitted for cancer treatment.

I tried to take several deep breaths and focus.

"I really can't think what my choices might be."

"There's Dana Farber in Boston, Dartmouth Hitchcock in Hanover, New Hampshire, and Maine Children's Cancer Program in Portland, Maine," she said.

"What are the differences between them? Is any program better than the others? I mean, I know Dana Farber and Dartmouth Hitchcock by reputation, but what about Maine Medical?"

"I know one of the doctors, Annie Rossi, a hematological oncologist, very well and the other doctors are from places like Children's Hospital of Philadelphia, St. Jude's, and Tufts New England. Even though the program has only been there for four or five years, it has a first-rate reputation, and all of the physicians are excellent. You do understand Hannah needs to be hospitalized as soon as possible."

"Yes, yes, of course I do."

Unable to figure out how to decide, I seized on the difficulty of getting there. Dartmouth was over two hours away. Boston and Portland were each about an hour away, but driving into Boston in the best of circumstances was difficult. A decision had to be made. Hannah urgently needed to be somewhere for treatment.

I tried twice before I found my voice.

"I guess we'll go to Maine Medical Center."

I didn't hear anything else of the conversation. Words, images, sounds flashed through my head, all of it chaos. Only one image was clear: Hannah had cancer. My safe, normal world lay around me in ruins.

Chapter 2

AMERICAN FAMILY

A house, two point five kids and a dog.

U ntil the moment I heard Hannah's diagnosis, I had considered us a normal American family. My husband, Mike, and I met at the University of New Hampshire where he was doing his Ph.D. in electrical engineering. At the time, I had just started my own practice as a Nurse Practitioner in York, Maine. To supplement my practice income, I treated patients at the University of New Hampshire Student Health Services two days a week.

On those days, I ate at the Memorial Union Building. It was always overcrowded, so sharing a table with someone you didn't know was common. One Tuesday as I was working on a seminar I was preparing to teach, a man's voice asked about sharing my table. Without glancing up, I nodded assent. Then, a pair of very long muscular legs caught my eye. As I scanned upwards, I saw they were attached to a very good-looking guy. Trying not to stare, I put my eyes back on the work I was doing as he sat down opposite me. Conversation wasn't the rule in these situations, but he leaned across the table and asked what I was working on. I explained about the workshop and that I saw patients at the Student Health clinics, and asked what he did at the university. He told me about his Ph.D. program and work.

As I reluctantly got up to leave, he said, "My name's Mike. Do you eat here every day?"

"No, I'm only here on Tuesdays and Thursdays and my name is Carol."

Our romance began. It has lasted through a happy marriage and the blessing of our lives with two daughters, Caitlin and Hannah.

While Mike was finishing his degree, he designed computer software for a local high-tech start-up, and stayed on after he graduated because he liked being close to home and loved the work. After ten years, when that company failed, he took a position with a telecom start-up in Massachusetts.

I had enjoyed my fifteen years in private practice before my children were born and when they were small. But with Mike working an hour away and both girls entering new schools, I decided to leave my practice to be a full-time mom. I had never before not worked, but I selfishly enjoyed the luxury of devoting my full attention to my daughters' journeys toward adulthood and pursuing my own interests in writing, gardening, and sewing.

Caitlin, who was shy, had found the transition from middle to high school difficult, but Hannah, who had always been much more outgoing, made the change from elementary to middle school with ease. She loved her teacher and their fifth grade classroom was a lively, exciting place to be. A salmon fish hatchery occupied one corner, colorful poster presentations jockeyed for space on the walls, and lively discussions of raising fish to release into a local stream was a part of all their class work.

She couldn't wait to go to school each day, and despite a full schedule of travel soccer, dancing on toe in ballet, and studying classical piano, she never seemed to tire. When she wasn't involved in one of her many activities, she did what she loved to do best--read books. Her wry sense of humor helped her handle most situations with a grace and ease belying her age. Her teachers described her as a great asset in the classroom, an enthusiastic learner who was always willing to help other students.

Coaching girls' soccer lit up Mike's life. He loved teaching, not the skills so much, but how to be a team member. He had started when Caitlin was in kindergarten and had advanced to travel soccer coordinator while continuing to coach a travel team. With a van to prove it, I was a soccer mom and super fan on the sidelines. Weekends involved away travel or home games and sometimes both. Caitlin and Hannah were best friends and our trips to various events were full of laughter and play. We liked being together and felt blessed with a rich and happy family life.

Chapter 3

FOREWARNING

Prodrome: symptoms indicative of impending disease.

I had to consciously unclamp my hand from the phone to put it down. I thought about what had happened to our lives in the last few minutes. That family had been who we were, but not anymore. The events of the last five months ran through my mind. All the symptoms were clear and obvious. Each of the changes in Hannah's health, which at the time had seemed to be isolated problems, now clicked into place forming a picture I hadn't been able to see. I was a good diagnostician, but I hadn't recognized it. A million what-ifs ran through my mind.

My confidence was shaken, but at the same time I thought, *Why hadn't anyone else considered leukemia? Why had I had to fight and demand to get a workup and blood work if she was this ill? Would they have even done the workup if I hadn't known that she needed it?* Now, of course, I had the results I'd demanded and I didn't want them. I wanted to beg for some other answer; I wanted the doctor to be wrong, but I knew she wasn't.

My thoughts went back to December when Hannah had developed what had turned out to be a viral infection. We had been particularly busy because, even though soccer slowed down to weekend indoor games in the winter, swimming and ballet were in full season. Caitlin had club swim meets, high school swimming, and school finals, while Hannah had rehearsals for the *Nutcracker* ballet, piano, and indoor soccer. With ballet performances the week before Christmas and celebration of Hannah's birthday three days after, we were in overdrive.

After her birthday, Hannah, who had always been very healthy and rarely was ill with anything other than a cold, developed an unusual rash on her chest, neck, and stomach. I took her to the doctor to make certain it was nothing serious. The physician who saw her felt it was probably a virus, but at my insistence did blood work. When the tests came back, my worry seemed unfounded as they showed it was, in fact, caused by a virus. Thankfully, she recovered and soon was back to her normal activities. I hadn't thought about it again until now. Could this virus have "broken" something when it used her body to replicate its RNA? Could that have been the beginning? There wasn't any way to know.

More memories of episodes in the last few months came to mind. With a shiver, I remembered what I now felt had probably been a premonition. On what seemed an ordinary day earlier in the spring with nothing on my mind other than the chores for the day, I started my shower. Midway through, with no warning, the image of losing my whole family filled my head. The vision was so real, so vivid; I began to sob and shake. Barely able to stand, I leaned against the wall tiles doubled over in pain. Shampoo and water ran down my face mixing with my tears, and choking sobs made it hard to breathe.

Fumbling for my towel, I wrapped it around me and sat on the floor until I could stop crying. There was no logical explanation for such an intense feeling of loss and desolation. Everyone seemed okay. Mike's work was going well; the girls were fine and doing well in school. I didn't have any health concerns and nothing else I could think of would explain such an awful thought. I rationalized that I might be overtired, or having a flashback to a few months earlier and the terrible events of 9/11, or maybe it was changing hormones. By the end of the week, the feeling was nearly forgotten, but every once in a while, when I was having a bad day, that feeling of impending loss and doom would nag at me.

In mid-March we traveled to Hanover, NH, for Caitlin's swim team championships. Hannah and Mike joined us on Saturday after the indoor soccer game. She was so tired at dinner that she almost fell asleep in her plate. Since she slept most of the way in the car as well, I was concerned that she was getting sick again. She didn't have a fever, and wasn't complaining of feeling sick to her stomach or any other flu symptoms. After a night's sleep, she seemed much better. I figured it must be a twenty-four-hour bug, she might be growing again, or she was just overtired from all of her activities.

I stared blankly at the work I had been doing before the phone call, thinking about all the little things that had led to her diagnosis. I was second-guessing myself about not being able to diagnose her. While my worry about her was constantly in the back of my mind, Hannah hadn't complained, kept up with her activities, and did well in school. Should I have insisted on more testing sooner?

The first really serious thing had been her jaw pain in mid-April. As she sat down to breakfast one morning before school, she said, "Mom there's a lump right here on my jaw that hurts."

"How long have you had it?"

"I noticed it yesterday and then this morning it really hurt."

I felt the lump on the right side of her lower jaw and looked into her mouth. There wasn't any swelling or redness and her teeth looked fine.

"It's probably your braces. Your appointment's next week. Let's have the orthodontist check it then. Okay?"

She agreed and didn't mention it again. At the time, I assumed I was correct; now I knew how wrong I had been.

We had seen the orthodontist as planned. She took X-rays and found an area of missing bone immediately above the sore spot. She didn't know exactly what had caused it and wanted us to see our regular dentist to have the tooth evaluated, thinking it might be an abscess.

I called our dentist, but unfortunately he was going to be out of town the next week and wasn't able to see her. He recommended an endodontist (a specialist who deals with the tissues surrounding the root of a tooth), and made the referral for the following Tuesday. In preparation, the orthodontist needed to remove the right lower side of her brace appliance on Monday.

During the weekend, Hannah went to bed early and didn't seem very hungry, but told me she didn't feel bad in any other way. I assumed that the lump was probably from an infection. After the removal of her braces on Monday, the orthodontist was more concerned and called a local oral surgeon. He agreed to see Hannah after lunch. After he looked at the X-rays and examined Hannah, he felt she should still see the endodontist the next day. He also hadn't seen anything like this before and recommended a bone biopsy if the tooth was viable and there wasn't an infection. I didn't like what a biopsy implied, but it all seemed a medically reasonable approach.

The endodontist insisted on seeing Hannah without me in the room. I waited impatiently in the reception area picking up various magazines, but unable to focus long enough to read anything. When he finally opened the door, I stood up so suddenly, I dropped my purse and the magazine from my lap. He ushered Hannah out into the waiting room and motioned me to come in.

"Are you okay?" I asked as I quickly hugged Hannah.

She put her head on my shoulder for just a second and hugged me back and said, "I'm okay, Mom."

She didn't sound very convincing to me, and as I walked into his office, I kept glancing backward to assure myself she was indeed okay by herself as she sat down to read her book.

"She doesn't have an infection and the tooth is viable, but I can't explain the missing bone. She needs a bone biopsy. Do you have one scheduled?" he asked.

"We saw the oral surgeon yesterday and he recommended one. I'll call him today and schedule it."

His brusque, hurried manner didn't invite questions and my mind was nearly blank. I couldn't think of anything else to ask, so I thanked him, collected Hannah, and headed for the car, trying to ignore the churning in my gut.

I put my arm around her, and then teasingly said, "Well, buggy, buggy, you need a biopsy to see what's going on with your jaw."

"Will it hurt? This thing to test my tooth kinda hurt."

"I'm so sorry it hurt and I couldn't be there to hold your hand. You were very brave to be in there by yourself. Are you okay now?"

She nodded.

"You'll be asleep for the biopsy and won't feel anything."

"That'll be weird. I've never had anything like that before."

I assured her it would be fine and I would be with her.

During the drive home, her concerns apparently forgotten, she chattered about what she was going to do the rest of this April vacation week. I listened with half an ear, absently mumbling appropriate responses to her plans while trying to puzzle through possible sources of her symptoms. I didn't like the direction this was taking; the biopsy appointment couldn't come soon enough. Unfortunately they didn't have anything sooner than two weeks away on Friday, May 10th. Hoping for a cancellation, I asked to be put on the waiting list.

The next day Hannah woke up with right ear pain. We headed back to Kittery to the doctor's office and while she was being examined I explained about the bone defect, since it was on the same side. The doctor didn't feel it was likely that there was any connection between the two. An antibiotic would take care of the ear infection, but he was certain the lump was still probably related to her braces in some way.

She went back to school the following Monday, excited about the scheduled salmon release later in the week. All she cared about was being there for that. I wanted her to be able to participate, but also kept hoping they would move the date of the biopsy appointment forward. I was trying to balance her desire to take part in the finale of their special project with my needing to know what had caused the lump.

Now, thinking back to that time, I knew that if I had seen her through a health care provider's eyes, not having seen her daily as my child, she would have looked sick to me. I was too close to be objective; seeing her every day, the subtle changes weren't as obvious. Had I viewed video taken at the salmon release or known she hadn't been telling me how bad she really was feeling because she didn't want to miss any soccer, ballet, or school, I would have insisted on more testing sooner. As it was, I didn't, but my worry about her was the white noise in my mind as I did spring cleaning, put in my vegetable garden, and dealt with the daily ups and downs of family life.

Remembering the last two weeks, everything seemed to have happened quickly and yet it felt as if it had been in slow motion.

In the middle of the night on the Monday before the Friday biopsy appointment, Hannah's crying woke me. She complained of a sharp, burning pain under her right shoulder blade. I examined her and couldn't find anything wrong. She wasn't having trouble breathing, her shoulder and arm were fine, and she didn't have a fever or nausea. I gave her some ibuprofen and she went back to sleep. She had played goalie in the weekend soccer game and had been run into a couple of times, so I assumed she must have twisted her back somehow. The next morning she said she was fine, but now her unexplained shoulder and back pain was added to my accumulating store of worries.

On the night before her biopsy, I realized my fears were greater than I was even admitting to myself. While I was fixing supper, Hannah was lying on the floor doing her homework, listening to one of her favorite CDs, the sound track from *Lord of the Rings*. As I bent over the oven to take out the casserole I'd baked, the horrible thought, *We'll have to be sure to play this at her funeral* came unbidden into my mind. I was barely able to set the casserole on the stove before I doubled over in pain. Tears rolled down my face and I fled upstairs so that Hannah couldn't see me crying.

I sat on the bathroom floor staring into space and trying to take deep breaths. Were we going to lose everything that mattered? Adding up all that had happened from the lump on her jaw, the grave attitude of the endodontist, her ever-increasing fatigue, and her decreasing appetite, I thought this could all be a part of some type of bone cancer, but until we had the biopsy results, I was helpless to do anything except wait and worry. I felt like screaming, but instead I bathed my face in cold water and went downstairs to serve supper.

At the oral surgeon's office, as we waited for them to do the biopsy, I thought that once we knew the source of her problem, it could be fixed.

How wrong I was.

As we sat side by side in the waiting room, Hannah looked up from her book and asked, "Do you dream when you have anesthesia?"

"I don't know if everybody does, but I've had some wonderful 'living in another world' dreams when I've had it. Why? Are you worried?"

"No, I just wondered what it's like."

"You won't feel anything once you're asleep, and when you wake up, you probably won't remember much about it," I assured her.

She grinned and went back to her book. I snuggled her close to me, kissed her forehead, and tried to match her relaxed approach as I prayed that all would go well, and she would have wonderful dreams.

Neither of my children had ever needed surgery, and watching Hannah in the surgery suite as she played around with the chair and giggled a lot, I thought about all the children I had cared for in my nursing experience. All those times I'd taken someone else's child to the operating room was a totally different experience from leaving my own child alone under anesthesia. Once she was asleep, I resisted the urge to hover outside the door and reluctantly returned to the waiting room, where my unread book occupied my lap and thoughts of all that could go wrong occupied my mind. When they finally told me she was waking up from anesthesia and doing well, I let out a huge sigh. Only then did I realize how much of that hour had been spent holding my breath.

Before going into the recovery area, I met with the oral surgeon, who explained what he had found.

"The biopsy went really well, but I've never seen a piece of bone just flake off like that. I'll send it out to pathology, but I still don't know what caused this to happen."

"No idea at all?"

"None. Whatever it is, it's unusual."

"When will you have the results?"

"For certain, it should be back by the time she has her follow-up appointment in a week."

"If you get results sooner, will you call me?"

"We certainly will. You can take Hannah home as soon as she wakes up enough."

I thanked him, made the follow-up appointment, and walked to the recovery area to sit with Hannah while she came out of anesthesia. Even though I was relieved she was okay after the surgery, I felt my spirits sag. This wasn't the definitive answer I'd wanted; this wasn't resolution, just more ambiguity. Intellectually I knew medicine was like this, but I wanted definitive and immediate answers.

Hannah insisted the following Monday that she was fine, ready to go back to school. I reluctantly agreed and convinced myself she would slowly regain her energy. Soon we would have the results from the biopsy and know the cause of the bone loss which would be something benign.

Soon we would look back on this and laugh at our fears.

During that long week, not only weren't my hopes realized, but in fact by Wednesday Hannah was more pale and tired than she had been. She still went to dance, soccer, and other school activities, but no matter what the results of the biopsy were, she wasn't regaining her strength and energy.

When we saw the oral surgeon for her postoperative follow-up, my hopes rose again when he reported what he had found.

"She's healing fine. The pathology report indicated this was fibrous dysplasia, which is part of a group of conditions in which normal bone is replaced with fibrous tissue leaving a defect in the bone. It's the most common benign bone tumor."

As he said the magic word *benign*, I breathed a sigh of relief.

"Why would Hannah have something like that happen? Is it related to her having grown five inches over the last year and trying to grow her jaw with the braces?"

"It could be, but I really don't know. I'll call a pediatric endocrinologist to find out and let you know as soon as I get the information."

I was so relieved that bone cancer seemed to have been ruled out that I let myself take a deep breath and relax for the first time in three weeks. Hannah insisted she wanted to go back to school for the rest of the day. I also wanted to talk with her teachers about what we knew. Both her teacher and the classroom intern were happy to see her back in class and to hear that the biopsy results were benign. However, they had some concerns I hadn't been aware of. Her class participation had been decreasing along with her interest in helping other kids; she had even begun to put her head down on her desk at the end of the day.

This news wasn't good, but with the biopsy results and my fear of bone cancer gone, I tried to convince myself she would slowly return to her old self. We just needed to be patient and all would slowly resolve.

However, the end of that week dashed those hopes. At the soccer game on Sunday, she started to cry, and asked to come out of the game in the first part of the second half. Her side hurt and she was having trouble catching her breath. Hannah was a tough competitor who didn't like being out of any soccer game. There had to be something else wrong, but she insisted on Monday morning that she was fine to go to school.

When I picked her up from her piano lesson after school, she ate her snack, finished her homework, and then didn't want supper. Since she loved to eat, I checked her for a fever or other symptoms, but nothing else seemed to be wrong. She insisted she was just tired and wanted to sleep. I went to bed early as well, but slept fitfully struggling through unremembered, vivid dreams. When I woke on Tuesday morning all the worry of the last weeks was no longer in the back of my mind, but foremost. I wanted to pull the covers up over my head and not have to face the day. My new companion, a constant feeling of dread, sat dead center on my chest like a lead weight.

Mike and I had always joked that he was in charge of fun and I was in charge of work and worry. We actually complemented each other nicely because he worked very hard and worried about many things, but for the most part I was the queen of worry. Over the past few weeks, we had talked a lot about what might be going on with Hannah, but both of us had been positive that if the problem could be identified, a solution could be found. He trusted my clinical knowledge and felt if something truly bad was happening, I would figure it out. I had always trusted my diagnostic skills, but I had never tried to diagnose anything really serious with my own child.

As I sat on the side of the bed watching Mike get dressed for work, I told him, "I don't want to be a mom anymore. It's just too hard."

He quickly came around the bed and pulled me into his arms. "You always worry too much. Don't assume the worst. It'll work out."

"I just can't figure out exactly what's wrong. No one who's seen her seems to think it's anything too serious, but something is wrong and I'm scared."

He hugged me again, and in a mock Jamaican accent, said, "Don't worry, be happy Mon!"

I wanted to believe I was overreacting, worrying over nothing, but my Mom's heart and Nurse Practitioner's head had begged to differ. (Later Mike told me he didn't really believe what he was saying, but he didn't want to give in to fear.) After soccer practice that night he had further evidence that things were not okay: Hannah had been unwilling to run at the beginning of practice and sat out at the end. After only a few bites of supper, she complained of feeling full and went to bed. Neither Mike nor I slept well.

The changes in Hannah began to increase rapidly. Wednesday morning when she came down to breakfast after her shower, she gave me a hug. As I held her close, I noticed something I'd been bothered by a couple of times previously: she smelled ill. Having been around many patients with different illnesses, each with its own unique odor, she smelled like some kind of cancer. I hadn't said anything, but after she left for school, I wasn't able to focus on any of the things I had to do; the thought that she still might have some form of cancer ate at me. Worrying left me staring into space in the middle of a task, tears in my eyes and a grapefruit-sized lump in my throat. I was certain now that I wasn't overreacting, but until we got some more information from the pediatric endocrinologist there didn't seem to be anything else to do.

When she got home from school, she was upset because she had done badly in the Bagel Challenge. As a part of the fifth grade spring physical education program, they ran a 1.2-mile race each week. Our local bagel shop offered coupons to students who improved their times. The students were very excited about the competition and improving was really important to Hannah. She told me she had to stop and walk, and felt really bad about not doing well. Without any belief in what I was saying, I assured her she would do better the next time. Despite being tired, she insisted on going to dance class. With misgivings, I let her go.

When the carpool dropped her off, she dragged into the house complaining of her legs hurting and having trouble catching her breath when dancing.

"I think you should stay out of school tomorrow and I'll get you another doctor's appointment."

"Mom, I'm just tired. I don't want to miss school and we have soccer practice for the tournament. I need to go."

"I know you don't want to miss practice, but if they don't find anything, you can come back and go to practice."

"No, Mom. I just need some sleep."

I knew she wanted to be ready for the Memorial Day Tournament in Nashua on the weekend. Teams from all over southern New Hampshire, as well as Connecticut, Maine, and New York, would be there. It was exciting for the players and coaches to be in a big tournament and she didn't want to miss it. In retrospect, I should have followed my gut instincts, but instead I gave in again and let her go.

We had been very busy with preparations for the weekend and arrangements for Caitlin, since she had a swim meet and wouldn't be going with us. Our evening schedule was packed: soccer for Hannah and Mike, swim team practice and her spring school concert for Caitlin. And it was my turn to pick up the soccer practice carpool from school. I sat in the car waiting for dismissal, and as the line moved forward, I spotted Hannah with a teammate. Hannah was bent over, crying and grimacing with pain as she walked slowly toward the car. I started to get out, but by then she had climbed in and doubled up into a ball in the front seat.

"My back hurts again. I'm sick and my side hurts."

My patience for waiting to find out what had caused this came to an end. I called the doctor's office and spoke with one of the nurses I knew well. After listening to the brief history I gave her, she agreed Hannah needed to be seen. I quickly arranged for Caitlin to stay at school, since she needed to be there for the concert anyway. Mike was already at the soccer field, so I drove there, dropped off Hannah's teammate and talked with him about what had happened. He wanted to go along to the doctor's office, but needed to stay with the team to run practice. Since Hannah and I would already be in Kittery, we agreed to meet later at Caitlin's concert at Berwick Academy.

Every detail of the last twenty-four hours kept replaying in my mind. When the nurse checked Hannah in, she noted that her weight had dropped seven pounds since she was seen for her ear infection not quite four weeks before. I knew she hadn't been eating as much as usual and seemed to get full easily, but the loss of seven pounds was a lot. My mind kept going over and over the last few weeks as we waited to be seen. When the doctor, who was new to the practice, came in to examine Hannah, she acted annoyed with my request to have Hannah seen as an urgent appointment. Her tone of voice implied I was overreacting to something that wasn't a pressing problem. Was I really being unreasonable about the events of the last few weeks? I didn't think so.

After the third repetition of my concerns about the sequence of events since discovering the lump on her jaw, I began to feel like a broken record. My litany of events was that Hannah had been consistently tired, had lost a lot of weight for a healthy athlete, the pain under her shoulder blade had returned and was much worse, and she had almost completely lost her appetite. Even though I had been seeing her every day, she was pale, had deep, dark circles under eyes, and looked really ill. Had I been seeing her as a patient, I would have been very concerned.

As the doctor began to downplay my concerns, my frustration and rage suddenly took over, and I furiously spat out, "I want a workup! I want blood work with a CBC and differential, a chem. panel, and whatever else will look at what is causing her symptoms. I also want a chest X-ray to see why she has pain under her shoulder blade."

Whatever denial, fear, and inability to use my professional knowledge had kept me from recognizing what needed to be done was swept away in that outburst. My daughter was steadily getting sicker; what this doctor thought about me didn't matter, she needed to find out what was wrong with Hannah.

She replied, "Uh, okay. We should add a thyroid panel because of the weight loss and fatigue. Come in tomorrow morning. Our lab's already closed tonight."

Disgusted, I just nodded, put my arm around Hannah, helped her off the exam table, and left.

In the car, I steamed; Hannah doubled up in a ball, lay down and closed her eyes. I drove, muttering inside my head, angry and embarrassed that I had been treated as if I were some hysterical, overprotective mother. Something was seriously wrong with Hannah. We needed to find the source of her symptoms and I wasn't going to stop. If the mechanisms for ordering what she needed had been available to me, I would have done it myself.

Coming all the way back to Kittery in the morning didn't seem reasonable. They would need to send the lab work out and that would mean further delay. For the second time in one day, I used my cell phone while driving and called back to the doctor's office to tell them I wanted the testing done at Wentworth Douglas Hospital, preferably tonight. They told me the outpatient lab was already closed, and would reopen at 7 A.M.; the only choice would be the ER. I agreed to wait, not wanting Hannah to have to sit in the ER for a long time.

At Berwick Academy, Mike was waiting in the parking lot. I gave him an abbreviated version of events, not trusting myself to start telling him about it without upsetting him and Hannah. I felt bad about missing Caitlin's concert, but Hannah was too tired to stay.

Once we got home, Hannah wasn't feeling as bad, the pain was gone, and she even managed to eat some supper. I wanted it to be morning so the blood work and X-ray could be done and (hopefully) we would have an answer. Even though I knew deep down that any plans for the next few days probably wouldn't happen, some part of me still clung to a shred of hope that somehow, some way this would be resolved, allowing us to return to our normal lives.

After Mike and Caitlin got back, we talked about the concert and their worries about Hannah, and then went to bed. Mike and I lay awake reliving the day as I vented to him about the appointment, my anger and fears. Eventually exhaustion took over and we slept, only a few precious hours of innocence left.

Chapter 4
SOLVING THE PUZZLE

Diagnose: To determine the cause and nature
of a pathological condition; to recognize a disease.

Awakening at my usual 5 A.M., I wasn't able to get back to sleep. Wanting to get there when the lab and outpatient X-ray opened at 7:00, I completed as many chores as I could before waking Hannah.

Mike sleepily asked me, "Why do you want to get her up so early? Wouldn't it be better to let her sleep as long as she likes?"

"Maybe, but I'm really scared. The sooner we have the tests, the sooner we'll have results."

"Could she just not be sleeping well and with all that's happened, just need more sleep?"

"I don't think more sleep is going to solve this problem. Plus, I'm worried because it's the start of the holiday weekend and there might be reduced hours or services if she needs more testing."

Mike might have been correct about needing sleep, but the medical side of me and my mother's intuition told me we were past hoping for some simple, benign explanation of her symptoms. Time seemed crucial to me and I wanted the blood work and X-ray results.

Once we were at the hospital, I stood in line at the outpatient check-in so we could file the appropriate paperwork. Hannah leaned heavily against me. She'd been up for less than an hour and she was already pale and stooped with fatigue.

"Do you need a wheelchair, sweetie?"

With a deep sigh, trying to straighten up a bit, she said, "No. I'm fine, Mom. Let's just go get this done."

We walked slowly along the hall toward Outpatient X-ray. After checking in there, I helped Hannah put on a gown. Tears stung my eyes as I watched her gamely get ready for the X-ray. Over the last couple of weeks, she had become somewhat of an expert at medical tests and procedures. With a momentary flash of humor, she looked down at the hugely oversized blue gown and giggled. I tried to laugh, but instead busied myself with the string ties so she wouldn't see my tears.

The technician showed her how to stand at the machine for two films of her chest (front and side views). Putting on a lead-lined apron so I could be in the room, I stood watching her, my heart aching. It only took about five minutes, but as soon as she was done, she sat down heavily on the bench and leaned forward, breathing hard. I helped her dress and put my arm around her waist to support her as we left the X-ray area.

What athletic eleven-year-old used to running races, playing soccer, and dancing ballet gets out of breath changing her clothes? What was causing this? My mind was going round and round with unanswered questions, but still I couldn't see it. We had a negative biopsy report, none of the doctors seemed concerned, and nothing much had shown up on her examination. What was causing her symptoms to progress so rapidly in such a short time?

We trudged toward the outpatient laboratory waiting area. As soon as we reached a couch, she dropped onto it and when I sat down next to her, she sagged against my shoulder. I put my arm around her and held her close. No words came to me; there was nothing to say. Unable to find any way to vent my fear and frustration, I focused on how annoying it was to wait. Those twenty minutes could well have been hours.

When our name was finally called, I helped her into the blood draw area. Afraid she wouldn't be able to stay upright in the chair, I sat down first and pulled her onto my lap.

After filling the first tube, the technician looked at her and asked, "Are you okay? You look really pale. You're not going to faint on me are you?"

Hannah shook her head no, but slumped back against my neck. I caught, out of the corner of my eye, a glimpse of the tubes of blood lying on the counter. Expecting to see the deep, rich crimson of normal blood, I was shocked by the pale creamy liquid in the tubes. With no time to process what it meant, I worked on keeping Hannah propped up until the lab tech was done. I needed to get her home and then get these results. Whatever this was, it wasn't good.

I half carried her to the car. Once inside she put her seat back, lay down with a sigh, and closed her eyes. My palms were sweaty and my hands shook so hard, I fumbled with the key and after a couple of tries finally got it into the ignition. She looked so pale, so tired. My thoughts jumped from one symptom to the next; images flashing. My usual way of sorting and fitting data together to make a diagnosis was short-circuited by fear.

Gripping the steering wheel as if that would help me find an answer, I kept going over and over everything that had happened. Two days ago she had run a road race and danced for an hour; now she was ghostly white, unable to even sit up in the car. She needed to be back in bed, and I was glad I had followed my instincts about getting the tests done early.

While Hannah slept upstairs, I called Mike to let him know the testing was done.

"How'd it go?"

"She could barely sit up to have her blood drawn and I had to half carry her to the car."

"That doesn't sound good. She seems a lot worse just since yesterday. What are your thoughts?"

"That's the problem. I just can't get my mind around this. At this point, it doesn't add up. None of the doctors have suggested anything, so the lab results are what we need. I just want an answer soon."

"It'll be okay. We'll figure this out. Let me know as soon as you hear anything. I'll be out running at noon, but should be back by around one, so give me a call."

"I asked for everything to be stat, so hopefully we'll know sooner than that. I'll call the minute I get anything."

While I waited, I decided Hannah should probably try to eat something. I took her toast and scrambled eggs, and although she tried to eat, the effort was too much and she fell back to sleep after a few bites. I tried to go back to work on various tasks, but felt like a caged animal. Between efforts at completing paperwork, I paced or sat staring into space, my mind abuzz with questions. I tried to reason away my fear by reminding myself that none of doctors had been particularly concerned, no one had even suggested a diagnosis.

Every symptom was vague and non specific; no bruising or bleeding, no fevers, vomiting, or diarrhea, just fatigue, decreased appetite, weight loss, and the unusual back pain. Was it something like a thyroid disease, diabetes, or some other blood problem? The only specific thing was the fibrous dysplasia which was a benign result. Surely this had a simple explanation or it would be more obvious.

Like most parents, I figured out all kinds of minor things that went wrong with my children, but this was different. In the last couple of days with the return of her back pain and barely tolerating being out of bed for more than a few minutes, it was obvious she was getting sicker. There is a good reason medical personnel are discouraged from treating their own family members: their judgment isn't objective enough.

Looking back I think I was also in the grip of something I'll call "Mom Brain." Anyone who isn't a parent might find it hard to believe how much denial parents can be in when something happens with their child. While I had the advantage of medical knowledge, I was also seeing her every day and not actually seeing her. Emotional distance and objectivity weren't luxuries I had.

I checked on Hannah again and then forced myself to wait for the results, resisting the urge to call the office to see if they had an answer yet. Instead, I sat staring at the phone, willing it to ring.

Chapter 5

HURTLING TOWARD HELL
IN SLOW MOTION

I was sitting in the crater after the blast, shaking, ears ringing, head spinning and stomach churning. All the events of the past weeks fit seamlessly into a complete pattern. The memories of how we got to this point made me realize how much I had denied what was in front of me. I had a million reasons why that was true, but the weight of it bore down on me. There was so much to do and a new reality to come to grips with, but I couldn't get the phone call out of my head. I kept hearing the conversation over and over.

"Your daughter has cancer. Where do you want to go for treatment?"

So stark, so cold. There was no, "I'm sorry I have some bad news for you," not a word of consolation or support.

I couldn't imagine having to make such a call, but if I had to, I didn't think I would ever be so unfeeling. Was this because I had demanded the workup I thought Hannah deserved and in the process challenged this doctor's power? If a fellow health care professional was treated this way, how were others treated? What would it be like to have no knowledge of what was involved and be told this devastating news in an uncaring way? I was angry and felt like calling back and raging at this woman, but I knew I wouldn't. I had no control over this doctor's behavior; I only had control over how I helped Hannah survive. If she did, I hoped I wouldn't care, but for now it was the purest form of pain--a mother's fear for her child's life. At least I had my medical and nursing skills to fall back on as tools to help us get through this. Trying to get past my anger and upset, I forced myself to concentrate on the task at hand: getting Hannah to the hospital and treatment.

I had given approval for a referral without waiting to talk to Mike, because I wouldn't be able to reach him until 1 P.M., and I understood the urgency of her admission, and how sick she was. The sooner we got her into the hospital, the sooner they could begin treatment. Nevertheless, I needed to talk to Mike; and I had to explain to Hannah what was happening, and Caitlin needed to know. What was I going to say to each of them? How were we going to get through this? Would we survive, if she didn't? My shattered world lay around me like a valuable heirloom china plate; no matter how hard I tried, it would never be the same, there would be scars and cracks.

Now that I knew what was wrong with her, I wanted to un-know; I wanted to go back to March and do the last weeks over again. I wanted to rage at the gods and hide somewhere safe where this wasn't true. My child had cancer and she was getting worse by the hour; she could die if she didn't get treatment quickly. She could die even if she did get treatment. Being a health care professional hadn't been enough; education, success, nothing had made us immune from something terrible happening.

I tried again to reach Mike. No matter how bad I felt, he would be even more devastated. His daughters were the light of his life, and the thought that this was happening to one of them would be unbearable. I knew we would fight together for Hannah, but I felt he would rely on my professional skills to handle a lot of this. I would need to be an umbrella protecting us all, both a Mom and a Nurse Practitioner.

I gathered myself to go upstairs to talk with Hannah. Just as I was finally able to stand without my knees giving way, the phone rang again.

A warm, friendly voice said, "This is Dr. Schwenn. I'll be Hannah's oncologist." Her words stopped me cold. *Oncologist? How could my daughter need an oncologist?* I swallowed hard past the lump choking my throat and introduced myself.

"Hannah has a type of leukemia, which is a disease of the white blood cells. It is one of the cancers seen in children," she said.

As she began a lengthy, general description of what leukemia was, I realized she wouldn't have any way of knowing my background. When she asked if I had questions about what it was, I told her I was a Nurse Practitioner and asked for more specifics from the testing.

She immediately switched gears and said, "Hannah's white count is 35,000 [very elevated] with greater than 8% blast cells, which are indicative of leukemia. The X-ray showed an unexplained shadow around her right lung. Her platelet count is only 99,000. Have you noticed any unusual bruising?"

"No we haven't. What she has had is a pain under her right shoulder blade, loss of appetite, fatigue, and shortness of breath when she's been playing soccer or dancing. She's lost seven pounds in a little under a month and has been very pale. She also had a lump on the right side of her lower jaw which turned out to be benign fibrous dysplasia."

We continued to talk briefly about Hannah's symptoms, the types of leukemia, and childhood cancer in general.

"We don't know the exact type of leukemia at this point, but once you're here, we can begin the workup. I know this is really hard. I am so sorry you have to go through this, but I know you understand how sick she is and that this *is* a medical emergency. She needs to be here as soon as you can bring her. The traffic will be bad because of Memorial Day so drive carefully. Any more questions?"

"No, you answered most of my immediate questions. We'll be there as soon as we can."

One of the staff nurses came on the line and gave me instructions for the admission process and how to find the Admitting Department at Maine Medical Center. When I hung up the phone, I sat head in hands trying to process what I'd heard. Even though I was scared to death about Hannah and all Dr. Schwenn had told me, I was relieved she would be cared for by someone who sounded very competent, knew what needed to be done, and most importantly was in charge.

Thankfully, Mike answered on this third try to reach him. When I heard his voice, I fought not to cry. I was afraid if I started, I wouldn't stop.

"Are you sitting down?" I asked.

"Just tell me what it is."

"Hannah has leukemia. The blood tests don't show exactly what kind of leukemia it is. On the X-ray there is a shadow around her right lung, but they don't know what that means. They want her in the hospital immediately."

I could hear his voice catch as he asked, "What's the plan?"

I told him about the decision I had made about where to go. Then I repeated my conversation with Dr. Schwenn.

"As soon as I can, I'll get Hannah packed up and in the car and then pick up Caitlin at Berwick and head to the hospital," I said.

"Okay, I'll meet you at the hospital as quickly as I can."

It all sounded so mundane, like a litany of chores, but it was a way of coping with the unimaginable. We didn't talk about our feelings. What we hadn't said communicated volumes. We had to take care of the task at hand. We were parents and falling apart wouldn't help Hannah or Caitlin. We would talk later. We didn't have time for the emotions we were feeling. This was urgent. We were both strong and I hoped we could do what had to be done.

My next task seemed un-doable. I needed to explain to Hannah that she had leukemia and was being admitted to the hospital. I didn't know if I could sit down with her and say, "You have cancer and they don't know exactly what kind it is." I felt as if I would choke on the words. I knew I needed to prepare her for admission, but could I do that without telling her the details? I stood up, but my knees were so wobbly I sat back down. Finally, I began climbing the stairs to her bedroom, hanging onto the railings to steady myself. I paused in the doorway of her room and looked at her, then walked to the bed and crawled in beside her. Holding her tight, I buried my face in her silky, long blond hair. It was heartbreaking to think of her perfect young body, which had always been so healthy and athletic, being possessed by an unseen enemy. I tightened my hold on her, never wanting to let go.

"Mom, what's wrong?"

"The tests you had done this morning show that you are very, very sick and need to be in the hospital for them to find out exactly what's going on. We need to gather up the things you want to take with you so we can get there as soon as possible."

My voice caught as I nearly started to sob.

"Mom, are you okay?"

"I'm upset you're so sick and need to go to the hospital, but I know they'll take care of you and find out more about what's wrong so you can get better."

As I gathered my courage to explain what she had, she interrupted to ask if she could take Lovey Bear and some of her books with her. A relieved coward, I answered her immediate question with a resounding yes. Talking to some else's child, as a professional, I think I could have said it all, but this was my daughter. I couldn't make the switch; the words wouldn't come.

Because of the urgent need to get her to the hospital quickly, I focused on organizing the necessities while she pointed out which books she wanted and held tightly to Lovey Bear. He was a small white Gund polar bear which had been hers since infancy. As a baby she would suck her finger and hold Lovey cradled in her arms rubbing his fur whenever she needed comfort. I said a silent prayer that Lovey would carry her through all of the awful moments I knew she would now be facing.

After packing a bag with pajamas, toiletries, extra tee shirts, and stretch pants, I told her to rest until I had the car loaded and we were ready to leave. I packed my own bag and checked to make certain I had the insurance information. As I was gathering everything, I started dreading the next task: telling Caitlin. She needed to be told not to board the bus for swim practice.

I called Berwick Academy, and once I had assurance from the receptionist that Caitlin would wait for us in front of the Burleigh Davidson building, I sat on my bed. I hadn't been able to say what our family emergency was when she asked. I wasn't yet able to tell anyone else that Hannah had cancer. By not saying it, could I make it not true? For just a brief moment, I thought about curling up on my bed in a little ball and being unconscious so that I didn't have to know. However, that wasn't one of my "Mom" choices, so I wiped my eyes, blew my nose, washed my face in cold water, and went to help Hannah to the car.

As I drove, I tried not to think about how Caitlin would react. She had always adored Hannah, and their closeness was a gift I treasured. Hannah and I were both quiet as we headed toward South Berwick, she from the effort of walking to the car and me from fear and sadness.

I pulled into a parking space in front of the school and saw Caitlin waiting. She started down the stairs looking annoyed and gesturing "what?" with her hands. She couldn't see Hannah lying down in the front seat. I jumped out of the car and walked to her.

"Mom, where's Hannah and what's going on? Why am I not going to swimming?"

I pulled her to me and put my arms around her.

"Hannah's lying down. You know she went to the hospital for tests this morning. Well, the tests showed it's very bad. She's really sick. We're on our way to Maine Medical Center for her to be admitted to the hospital because she has cancer."

She stiffened in my arms, screamed, "NO!" and started to cry, yelling, "That's not fair! Hannah has never done anything wrong. She's a good person and she shouldn't have cancer."

My heart aching for both of my children, I held her, wanting to scream and cry along with her.

Instead I said, "I know that, sweetie, but we can't undo it. We just have to help her get through this. She's being admitted, so I couldn't let you go to swimming because I don't know when we'll get back tonight and I know Hannah will feel better if you're with her."

"Of course we're not going to the tournament this weekend. Dad's coming straight from work and he'll meet us there. Do you have all of your school stuff?"

She nodded her as she put her bags in the car. Still crying, she got into the car and immediately took Hannah's hand.

She said, "I am so sorry you have cancer. It's not fair!"

Hannah stared at her, looking puzzled, but continued to hold Caitlin's hand. I patted Hannah's arm and said, "I'm sorry."

My inability to say the word cancer to Hannah had come back to haunt me very quickly. I had said it to Caitlin, but still hadn't been able to say it to Hannah. Feeling as if my tongue were glued to the roof of my mouth, I couldn't find anything else to say. Negotiating traffic gave me an excuse not to talk or think.

Memorial Day weekend traffic going to Maine is the heaviest traffic of the year, and, worse, the Maine Turnpike was under construction. I wasn't happy to be driving in such bad conditions because I wanted to arrive as soon as possible, but another part of me was grateful because I didn't really want to arrive at all. I wanted to stop, or, better yet, reverse time to before all of this came into our lives.

As we crawled along in the stop-and-go traffic, the Oscar Meyer Weiner car, which is shaped like a big hot dog and bun, passed us. Hannah sat up to look and suddenly we were trying to remember the words to the Oscar Meyer Wiener song, but couldn't. It was such a silly thing to be laughing and worrying about the words to a commercial jingle when Hannah was so ill. It felt unreal and I kept waiting to wake up back in my own safe world.

As we sat waiting for traffic to move beyond another construction site, Hannah said, "Mom, you never told me I have cancer."

"I thought I may have mentioned leukemia when I was explaining about the hospital."

"I don't think so. I would have remembered that!"

"I'm sorry, sweetie. They don't know for certain yet exactly what you have. They think it is some type of cancer of the blood, but they still don't know exactly what's going on. The most important thing right now is to get you to the hospital where they can find out."

She gave me one of her deep thought stares, nodded and went back to resting and listening to music.

Nothing in my life had prepared me for this; not even the years of experience in my practice with patients and families were helpful. I felt guilty that I hadn't told her immediately, but I rationalized by telling myself that knowing wouldn't have prepared her for what was going to happen now. Not telling her went beyond believing that nothing like this could be happening. The word cancer is so loaded with negative, ugly meaning that telling someone they have it is terrifying. Perhaps, subconsciously, I thought it would be easier if she wasn't as scared as I was.

Hospitals were familiar territory. I usually walked into them as a professional, competent, decisive, at ease. I had been to Maine Medical Center for professional conferences and knew where it was. Now as I saw it perched atop the Western Promenade, it bore no resemblance to anything familiar. In a few minutes we were on Bramhall Street, where I could see the large blue "Admitting" sign. I spotted a parking space immediately in front of the entrance and thought, A*t least Hannah won't have far to walk.* Later, I thought about how I had handled this and realized how deep my denial was. Staff didn't park near entrances, and using a wheelchair hadn't been a thought. She was still my strong, healthy athletic daughter, not a dangerously ill child.

After I put the car in Park, I sat trying to take a couple of deep, calming, yoga breaths, but I couldn't. I wasn't ready for this, actually admitting her to the hospital. I put my feet on the ground, but my knees knocked together and my legs felt like jelly. I quickly sat back down pretending I had forgotten something inside the car so the girls wouldn't see how shaky I was. I had to help Hannah, so by a force of will I told my body to stop shaking and then walked around to her side of the car. I could function, but couldn't stop the inner trembling. Caitlin took our bags and I held onto Hannah as we walked into the hospital.

Chapter 6
LONG-TERM PARKING

*Hospitalization: to admit someone to the hospital
for treatment, diagnosis, or observation.*

I found a chair for Hannah and then fidgeted beside the information desk waiting for someone to escort us to the admission offices directly behind it. Hospital business bustled around us. Loudspeakers blared out pages for doctors and other personnel while patients in wheelchairs or on stretchers traveled to destinations unknown. Our unknown destination wasn't a place; it was somewhere in the future. As much as I suddenly hated hospitals, I needed this one which for now held the key to Hannah's survival.

As a health care provider, I created billing charges but didn't have to wade through the pounds of paper work involved in getting insurance approval. As I completed form after form, all I could think about was *this is supposed to be an urgent admission for a very sick kid.* There didn't, however, seem to be any way of rushing the insurance bureaucracy.

I honestly don't remember how long it took, but at one point a clerk requested that I move my car over into the long-term parking area across the street. As I hurried back, I thought, W*hat a prosaic metaphor that is. We have entered a realm defined by the concept of long-term parking.*

When I returned, Hannah was half lying on the settee in front of the giant fish tank in the reception area with Caitlin as her faithful attendant. I wanted to be done with this so she could lie down again in a bed. I tried to be courteous and pleasant, but it was hard to contain my increasing annoyance. Finally, the last form was signed, transportation arrived, and we were on our way to the inpatient unit.

The transportation aide brought a bariatric (oversized to fit extremely obese people) wheelchair. Everything we had with us, plus Hannah, fit into the chair, and I think Caitlin could have ridden as well. As Hannah sat doubled over amid the luggage, she looked like a white-faced china doll whose body had lost its stuffing. I held her hand and chatted with the transportation aide, again hoping that I could make this less frightening if I sounded positive about the whole process. As we waited for the elevator, Hannah looked trustingly up at me. Her eyes seemed to say that nothing could go wrong as long as I was there. I wished it were true, but I doubted I had any control over what would happen next.

As we got closer to the pediatric unit, I felt as if I were two different people. The medical me saw only the familiar, nonthreatening equipment, procedures, and staff, but to the Mom me, it all looked alien. I had shaky hands, wobbly knees, and a stomach ready to share its contents with the outside world. Worried that my emotions would cloud my ability to think clearly about what was happening medically, I tried to create a buffer from my fear. Twenty years of clinical practice had taught me to handle medical situations with my logical mind. I might have strong emotions, but being effective required thinking clearly at the time and handling the emotional impact later. My fear was threatening to undo me; I had to switch to professional mode.

The elevator stopped at the 6th floor of the L.L. Bean building, where we exited to the left up an inclined, windowed ramp. To the east was Deering Oaks Park, the Back Bay, and downtown Portland, and on the other side were the Western Promenade and the working harbor. It was a spectacular view, but I couldn't take my eyes off the heavy double doors of the pediatric unit straight ahead.

We crossed the threshold and I blinked in the bright lights of inpatient pediatrics. While other nurses I knew loved pediatrics, I had never liked caring for sick kids. Too many things could go wrong, and children couldn't always communicate what they were feeling. The transportation aide stopped at the main nurse's station directly ahead of us, where a clerk pointed us to the right toward a second nurse's station. I tried to reassure Hannah and distract myself by pointing out how nice everything was. The patient rooms we passed had large observation windows as front walls, many of which were painted with animal or cartoon-character scenes. Brightly colored curtains provided any needed privacy. Since the patient rooms were on the outside of the unit, each had its own window. It looked very nice, but at the moment I didn't care. Were they good at treating cancer? That was what mattered.

As we stood in front of the second nurse's station to turn in our paperwork, I had a feeling of dislocation. Usually I was on the other side of that desk, an insider. My role was to admit a patient and help his or her family feel cared for, to be knowledgeable and capable, and to help them cope with the terrible events they were facing. I could do this and go home at the end of the day satisfied I had made a difference. Now there was no end of the day. I couldn't go home from this. I was that person facing a terrible situation.

We were directed to the room immediately across from the nurses' station, a room for the sickest patients. It was big, filled with light, with lots of cabinet space and a couch under the double windows providing a view of downtown Portland. There was a beautifully tiled bathroom and the piece of furniture I was having trouble looking at, the bed. That place where they put sick patients, dying patients, suffering people. My heart hurt at the thought of who was going to occupy this particular bed.

The transportation aide unloaded our bags and started to help Hannah out of the wheelchair into the bed. I stepped in, thanked her, and took Hannah's arm. If Hannah had to be in this bed, I was going to be the one who helped her change into a gown and settle in. With a sigh of relief, she collapsed onto the bed. I hugged her and then she curled into a ball and closed her eyes as I covered her with the sheet.

I stood beside the bed looking down at her, seeing her in two ways at once. Clinically, I saw a child who could have been in a portrait entitled "Ill child." She looked sick, had a slight droop on the left side of her face, and was much too thin. My Mom's eyes saw too much white; her pale face and blond hair made too little contrast with the sheets and pillow. The only colors were the dark circles under her eyes and the blue-flowered gown that dwarfed her skinny body. Her normal vibrancy was gone. On the verge of falling apart, I turned away and began to put her things in closets and drawers. I desperately needed to have control over something in this room, and organizing her things was all there was.

Her rest didn't last long, as her nurse, Cathy came in, introduced herself, and began the admission. I felt relieved as I watched her interact with Hannah. Her smile was infectious and she made the whole process feel nonthreatening. She welcomed us to the Maine Medical Center (MMC) Pediatric Inpatient Unit, and said this section of pediatrics specialized in caring for children with cancer. She explained that this room and bed would be Hannah's space. Their policy was to avoid doing anything painful in the room since they wanted it to be a safe place for the child. Any procedures that could be painful would be done in the treatment room down the hall. She showed Hannah how her bed worked and how to operate the call system and television.

I had never truly realized, when we admitted a patient, how overwhelming the number of questions we asked could be. It was hard to even hear what was being asked, let alone assimilate it all. I understood why it was needed, but could barely cope with it. All I knew was that Hannah was now officially an inpatient in a cancer treatment facility.

That, of course, wasn't where the admission ended; she still needed a physical exam. In teaching hospitals, house staff, interns and residents are physicians in training. They learn a specialty by caring for hospitalized patients under the supervision of the medical school faculty and specialists who are actually responsible for the patient's care. Cathy told us a resident in Pediatric Oncology would be doing Hannah's exam.

A few minutes later, he entered the room and introduced himself from where he stood just inside the doorway. Without shaking hands with either Hannah or me, he began to speak loudly in a cold, condescending tone as he announced that he would be examining her. I wasn't certain whether he thought we were deaf, stupid, or both, but my hackles went up. Since he seemed about ready to start his exam without any explanation to Hannah, I walked over to the side of her bed and attempted to introduce myself. I told him a little about us and then assured him that Hannah would understand what needed to be done for the exam when he was ready to proceed.

He looked surprised that I had spoken, and also a little annoyed as he said, "Good, you know something. I won't have to talk down to you to make you understand."

I raised my eyebrows and made eye contact with Hannah. She shrugged, and although she cooperated with the exam, she didn't ask any questions and made no effort to hide her dislike. I suddenly had qualms about my decision to come here; if this was the quality of the staff, we were in the wrong place.

I took a step or two back from the bed, but continued to stand there as I answered his few questions as politely as I could. I didn't want to antagonize him in case he was going to be involved in Hannah's case, not wanting to risk compromising her care. Being in this situation was difficult enough without dealing with a doctor who didn't seem to give a whit about her. He completed a cursory exam and left without explaining any of his findings. I gave Hannah a quick hug and quietly fumed inside as she gratefully snuggled back down under the blankets. I thought again, *I hope we didn't make a mistake coming here.*

Feeling anxious and needing a moment away from seeing Hannah in bed too tired to even sit up, I stepped just outside her room and leaned against the wall. I indulged in a brief moment of fantasy imagining his pen leaking through the pocket of his starched white coat, or him slipping on a wet spot or experiencing some other dignity-losing event, but then decided I would rather just throttle him for treating Hannah as if she were beneath his consideration.

As I stood there trying to take a deep breath, Cathy walked over, gave me a hug and said, "I know this is really hard, but we will do whatever you need to help you through this."

I stiffened slightly, but then mumbled, "Thank you." The contrast with how we had just been treated was obvious. I relaxed my tight shoulders and was grateful that at least they had great nurses here. I thought, *I would have done exactly the same thing were I the nurse for a patient and family who needed a moment of reassurance after an uncomfortable experience.* It was a surprise to be on the receiving end of nursing support, but I knew how much I needed exactly that.

Able to take deep breaths again, I thought I was ready to walk back into Hannah's room, but as soon as I saw her lying so pale and still in that large hospital bed with Caitlin sitting beside her in a chair, I felt lightheaded, went to the couch, and plopped down. This was unreal. Yesterday at this time, I'd had no idea that we would be in a hospital facing an uncertain future. I felt as if I had slipped through a crack in the universe into an unknown world. The knowledge that I could never go back to the world that had been mine for so many years hit me with gut-churning force and I ran to the bathroom.

When I came out, Mike had arrived. It had taken much longer than he'd anticipated, since he was coming from Massachusetts and the traffic had gotten even heavier than when we had come through a couple of hours before. As I walked over to hug him, I couldn't look directly into his face, where his pain was so evident in his tear-filled eyes. I found his hand and held on as we stood side by side looking at Hannah lying in bed. I could feel his efforts to control the sobs that threatened to break through. I was afraid Hannah would be frightened if she saw us breaking down. I squeezed his hand, clenched my teeth, and swallowed hard to hold back my own tears. We had to be strong. He glanced at me and nodded. Hannah had to believe this was going to be okay and so did we. If we needed to cry, it would be away from her.

Mike hugged Caitlin and Hannah and then we sat on the couch while they watched TV. I filled him in on all that I had learned thus far. He had a multitude of questions for which, at this point, I didn't have answers. The problem was there *were no* definitive answers. Only time and more testing would give us the information we needed, and then it might be an answer we didn't want. I prayed Hannah would survive until treatment could begin. I couldn't even think about what might be involved in treating her leukemia, no matter what type it was. Focusing on immediate problems was not just the best coping mechanism I had, it was the only one.

Dr. Schwenn entered the room and introduced herself to us. As we stood to shake hands with her, I looked into the gentle, intelligent face of this graying, midforties woman wearing an ankle-length full skirt, a peasant blouse and Birkenstocks, and was immediately reassured that the impression I had received on the telephone was borne out in reality. However, as warm and caring as she was, she was also all business as she explained that everything needed to be done as quickly as possible.

"I am working on getting a surgical team to come in tomorrow so we can do a bone marrow aspiration and biopsy. We will take a sample of Hannah's bone marrow plus a tiny sample of bone so we can determine the exact type of leukemia. We are pretty certain from the blood tests that this is a type of myeloid cancer, but we don't yet know if it is acute or chronic myeloid leukemia. Her presentation is somewhat unusual and we need to do more testing."

"Can you treat both of those?" Mike asked.

"Yes, regardless of which type it is, neither one will be easy to treat, but there is a great deal of experience with treating them."

As she examined Hannah, she asked questions about our family history and got as much pertinent information about us as she could as we continued to discuss what would be happening over the next twenty-four hours.

The admission formalities were winding down. After a quick tour of the teen room next door, where there were comfortable couches and chairs, a video game station, a Foosball table, and a variety of board games, Caitlin was only interested in being with Hannah, content to watch a movie sitting in a recliner beside her bed. One of the staff showed Mike and me around the unit so that we would know where all of the facilities were. There was a family lounge with kitchen area, laundry, TV and computer, and full shower facilities. We were assured that we could keep extra food for Hannah in the nurse's station refrigerator and have access to food in the pantry. The solarium with its quiet nooks for reading or relaxing was beautiful. The attractiveness of the facility and all of the services that were available didn't make up for the fact that I still couldn't comprehend that we really had to stay here. I was still in shock, and although it was good that we would have what we needed while we were here with Hannah, all I could think about was what medically needed to be done next.

It was 8 P.M. on a day that seemed years long, and Hannah needed to sleep. Mike wanted to stay the night, since his work schedule during the coming week wouldn't allow him to be at the hospital as much as I could be. Worrying that none of the nurses could be as attentive as I would be, and that Mike wasn't as familiar with hospitals as I was, I hesitated about leaving. But I also knew how important it was to him to be there, so I agreed. I helped him make up the couch into a parent bed. With the back couch cushions removed and the addition of blankets and a pillow, it became a passable sleeping space. Although Mike's six-foot-five-inch frame didn't fit well on it, he wasn't concerned and assured me that he would be fine. Hannah's bed curtain at least provided some privacy.

I hugged Hannah and reassured her that her dad and the nurses would take good care of her. I reminded her to call the nurse if she felt at all bad or had any questions. Caitlin hugged her and then the two of us left for home.

Although I was not looking forward to the hour-and-a-quarter drive home, I knew that it would be a time for me to be with Caitlin to help her with what was happening. We didn't start talking until I had found the way back to the Maine Turnpike. The shock of her first question nearly caused me to drive off the road.

"Mom, did this happen to Hannah because I don't believe in God anymore?"

As she began to sob, I grabbed her hand.

"No, sweetie. That isn't why people get cancer. We don't know the cause of Hannah's cancer, but I don't think this is about punishment. Don't you think if God wanted to punish you for not believing, he would have given *you* cancer?"

"Well, maybe," she said, as she laughed and cried at the same time. "But Hannah doesn't deserve this, she's a really good kid and she never did anything to anyone else, so why should she have to suffer? Do you know that she has those glow-in-the-dark stars above her bed and that the big middle star is for God and all of the smaller stars around it are angels?"

I knew about the stars, but I didn't know she had that symbolism for them.

"No, I didn't know that and yes, you're right, Hannah doesn't deserve anything bad. I don't know why this happened. I have to believe that there's some reason, but I don't know what it is and maybe won't ever know."

"It's just so unfair that there are bad people and nothing like this happens to them."

"It seems that way, doesn't it. I've always believed that we don't get to decide those things, though. We don't have any way to know what someone that I decide is bad, may really be going through."

"Well, I just know it's wrong Hannah's so sick! She's just a kid and didn't do anything to deserve being in the hospital. This stinks!"

I squeezed her hand.

"We just have to help her get through this. She's a really strong and courageous kid and I hope we all get through this okay. How do you think Hannah feels about it?"

"I don't know, Mom. She doesn't seem that scared to me."

"You may be right, but I can't imagine being eleven years old, in the hospital and feeling as bad as she does, and not being scared, can you?"

"Nope."

"She really looks up to you, so if you'll give her lots of support and encouragement, it'll help her to hang in there, okay?"

"Sure, Mom."

We rode in silence and as best I could, over the center console of our van, I hugged Caitlin and whispered a prayer of thanks that my children were such wonderful people. This feeling of being a team for Hannah made us closer. It was a gift given to me by this experience, and I gratefully accepted it. I didn't know it then, but Caitlin was on the verge of growing up overnight. She provided constant loving support to Hannah at the hospital, and without any questions became my helper at home, never once complaining.

By the time we arrived home, I was too tired to do anything but take care of the dog and brush my teeth before I fell into bed. I thought I would sleep deeply, but it came only in fits and starts. Repeatedly, I awakened from brief periods of oblivion, and for a millisecond couldn't remember why I felt so sad and afraid. With awareness came deep, aching pain as I remembered exactly what had happened and cried myself back to sleep.

During one of my bouts of lying awake crying, I thought again about my premonition. This had to be the source of that feeling. My brain buzzed with self-doubt questions. Could we have done anything sooner? Why hadn't I recognized the symptoms as they were happening? Why hadn't we done blood work at the end of April when she had the ear infection? Why hadn't I insisted sooner that we get a more complete workup? Was she going to make it through this, and if she did what would she be like? What if she didn't survive? Was there any way I could go on if she didn't make it? What would happen to all of us without Hannah?

At 5 A.M., unable to stay in bed any longer, I got up and took the dog out for a short walk in hopes of clearing my head. Caitlin had a swim meet scheduled for the whole weekend and I'd made arrangements for her to get a ride with another family since we would have been at the soccer tournament. Now, I wasn't certain how Caitlin felt about participating. We clearly needed to let some people know what was happening, but it was still too early to call anyone.

I woke Caitlin to ask her what she wanted to do. She felt that she really couldn't face anyone today and didn't feel like swimming. With exams coming up, she wanted to study and decided to stay home. Hannah would have her bone marrow biopsy today, if they were able to arrange it. It would probably be easier for Caitlin not to be there while Hannah spent the day having tests and procedures.

"I'll take care of calling about the swim meet once I get to the hospital, and I'll call you as we find out more."

I held her close, told her how much I loved her and said, "I'm sorry you have to be here by yourself, but I need to be with Hannah and Dad."

"I'll be fine, Mom. Give Hannah a big hug for me."

My heart was torn between the needs of my two children. Caitlin was being asked not only to handle her own responsibilities, but spend time coping on her own. Trying to be a mom in two places at once was wrenching, but where I would be going didn't feel like a choice.

Thankfully, there was less traffic even though it was still heavy for an early Saturday morning. As I drove, I tuned the radio to classical music. It provided the solace that I needed as I let the tears flow. By the time I arrived at MMC, I had cried enough to regain my composure and was ready to face the day.

At the patient and family parking lot, I gratefully paid my dollar and shouldered my load of books for Hannah and clothes for Mike. The convenient access and inexpensive cost were a blessing. The maze of corridors that wound past the gift/coffee shop, the business offices, and the entrance to the main cafeteria were confusing, but I quickly found the correct elevator. All of this was already starting to feel familiar.

However, as I approached the large double doors of the Pediatric Unit, I stopped. On the other side was a world I didn't want to be in. My heart began to pound and my chest constricted as I pulled open the door. Nodding to the staff at the main nurse's station, I resisted the urge to give up all dignity and run down the hall. Instead I speed-walked and prayed that Hannah hadn't gotten worse during the night and no one had let me know.

At the entrance to her room, I stopped short. She lay completely still, eyes closed, her blond hair in tangles on the pillow. For one brief second, the room spun as I fought the urge to throw up, feeling as if I had been kicked in the stomach. Then she opened her eyes and saw me.

"Hi, Mom."

I swallowed my fear, put on a smile, and sat down on the edge of her bed so I could hold her in my arms.

"How did you sleep?"

"Okay."

Mike came around the curtain and gave me a quick hug.

"We had a quiet night after you left. We watched a little TV," he said.

I saw the intravenous in her left hand and the IV pump on its pole next to her bed.

"When did they start your IV?"

"After you left, we went down the hall to the treatment room. I think it was really late."

"Did it hurt when they put it in?"

"No. They put some kind of cream on my hand and numbed it. But Mom, I was so tired when they were done, all I wanted to do was get back to my bed. Dad was talking to the nurse and I couldn't wait, so I walked back to my room with my IV pump on its pole. It wasn't very heavy, but it was so hard to push the pole that I didn't think I'd make it. That's probably the longest walk I've ever taken."

Aloud I sympathized with her while my heart started pounding again as I thought, *She is really deteriorating fast. She can't even walk twenty feet without feeling as if she might collapse.* I got up and busied myself putting away the clothes I had brought, showed Hannah which of her books I had in the bag, and chatted aimlessly about Caitlin and the dog.

Mike left to take a shower and get some breakfast. He didn't want to eat in front of Hannah, who would be NPO (nothing by mouth) until they decided if she would be having surgery. I cleaned up the parent bed area and neatened Hannah's bed. It would be a long morning while we waited to hear what the day would bring. I helped her get cleaned up and then couldn't sit still. She was content to doze, read, or watch television; I needed to be doing something. Reorganizing the drawers and cupboards in her room and setting up toiletries in the bathroom didn't help. We had been here less than twenty-four hours and time seemed to be standing still. Routines of meals, baths, tests, or procedures didn't do much to break up the day. I wanted to be at the next stage when we knew exactly what she had and if it would be treatable.

I tried to focus on just being there for Hannah, but was having difficulty. My association with patients in hospitals was having multiple people to care for, which meant being extremely busy every moment of the day. It also meant I felt as if I had some control over what was happening in their care. Waiting with nothing specific to do, not knowing what was planned next, and having no say in the situation was hard for me. I wanted there to be something I could do.

Chapter 7

GETTING TO THE
CORE OF THE MATTER

Bone marrow biopsy: surgical removal of tissue from the marrow of the bone for microscopic analysis and testing in the diagnosis of leukemia.

Mike and I waited for the doctors to make rounds so we could find out what was planned for the day. When they arrived, Dr. Schwenn explained she had, to her pleasure and surprise, easily assembled a surgical team to perform Hannah's bone marrow biopsy. She was delighted that on a major holiday weekend personnel simply respond with, "Sure, what time do you want me there?" We found throughout our stay this truly was the standard at MMC; patients came first.

Before the bone marrow biopsy, it was decided that Hannah needed a CT or CAT scan (computerized axial tomography), which would provide a 3-D picture of body structures (a regular X-ray is only two-dimensional). Because of the shadow seen on her chest X-ray and the pain in her back, they wanted to look at her lungs and the surrounding tissues. The Radiology Department was a busy place, especially on a holiday weekend with a large number of emergency room patients needing evaluation. So we sat waiting our turn, something we seemed to be doing a lot of.

When Hannah's name was called, the technician told us only one of us would be allowed to stay in the room with her while she was in the CT scanner. We both watched as she was injected with a dye which would allow them to see her lungs and upper abdomen better.

"You might feel a flush with a warm sensation like peeing your pants when the contrast dye goes in," the technician warned her.

Hannah giggled and looked at me. I smiled and squeezed her hand.

"That's so weird. Why does that happen?" she asked.

"It probably has to do with blood vessels reacting to the dye."

We watched the fluid as it flowed through her IV.

"Did it feel funny?" I asked.

Hannah laughed and said, "A little bit, but not bad."

Mike donned a lead-lined apron and stayed with her as I walked around anxiously in the waiting area. When they came out of the CAT scan lab, Hannah talked excitedly about what it was like with the clunking noise of the magnets as each slice of image was completed. She and Mike were deep into a technical conversation about how it all worked when the X-ray tech told her she needed another chest X-ray. She stood up for as long as it took, and then like a toy with run-down batteries, all her energy was used up. With her head on her arms, she sat waiting to be taken back to her room, where she curled up in bed completely spent from the half hour of effort.

She slept while we waited for them to take her downstairs for the biopsy. My mind was churning with what could go wrong in anesthesia and surgery. The thought that she could die from some complication of a test or procedure and not the cancer was unbearable. I forcibly put those images out of my mind so I wouldn't panic and follow my urge to grab her and run.

Finally we were back in the elevator going all the way down to the surgical suites in the lower basement. Instead of an operating room, we were taken to the large recovery room. They performed the bone marrow biopsies in one of the curtained cubicles. I tried to help Hannah relax by focusing on the decor. Disney and fairy-tale characters adorned the curtains and walls. At least they were trying to make it a nonthreatening, kid-friendly area.

Dr. Schwenn was there and introduced us to the anesthesiologist, who immediately tried to put Hannah at ease. He explained what he would be doing and told her if she went to sleep laughing, she would wake up laughing. She looked up at him with a question in her face as he drew the anesthetic into a syringe and then inserted the needle into a port on her IV tubing. Mike and I both squeezed her arm reassuringly and she settled back onto her pillow.

"Are you ready?" the anesthesiologist asked.

She looked up and nodded.

"Do you know why birds fly south in the winter?" he asked.

She looked intently at him and then shook her head and said, "No."

As he pushed the plunger on the syringe, he said, "Because it's too far to walk."

Hannah burst out laughing and fell asleep in mid-chuckle. Although she told me later she thought the joke was funny, she originally thought he was asking her some mental acuity test question to see if her brain was working okay. She had read somewhere that doctors tested patients that way. It made her nervous that he thought her brain wasn't working, so she was trying very hard to come up with the correct scientific answer.

As Mike and I returned to Hannah's room to wait, I tried to put the images of the biopsy procedure out of my mind. A large-bore needle would be inserted into her iliac crest (hip bone) to withdraw marrow (the soft center of the bone) and a bit of the bone for analysis. I knew she wouldn't feel it, but it wasn't a pleasant thought. Instead, I focused on what needed to happen next. This was the first time Mike and I had sat down together to talk and figure out how we were going to handle the next few days. We needed to make arrangements for Caitlin so she had rides to and from the school bus as well as swimming practice. Mike felt he really needed to be at work because he was very concerned about his job and the insurance end of the picture.

He told me he had called the human resources person at his company as soon as he received my phone call to ask about being covered for care at the Maine Children's Cancer Program, since we had Massachusetts insurance. She checked into it and gave the go-ahead, but we were still concerned. High-tech start-ups were great places to work if you were creative in software design like Mike was. However, since the high-tech bubble was in the process of disappearing, there had been a lot of closures in the last few months. This meant the future was never very certain, and although his company seemed to be okay for now, our worries continued.

As I repeatedly straightened and reorganized Hannah's room, I resentfully thought about health insurance issues. While we were terrified Hannah would die, we also had to waste energy worrying about our health insurance. Loosing coverage was scary even if you were healthy, but if you had a preexisting condition, it was a disaster. If she survived and we didn't lose insurance while she was in treatment, she would definitely have a preexisting condition and we might never be able to get insurance coverage for her again. If she had ongoing treatment needs, we could be bankrupt.

In America one of the most common causes of personal bankruptcy is a medical problem that just wipes out everything you have. Once again I had to separate myself from a problem I couldn't solve and focus only on things I could do something about. For now we still had coverage. Disaster would have to wait for the future.

There was so much to be taken care of. The soccer team was surely wondering what had happened to their coach and one of their key players. We needed to keep in touch with family and the school needed to know that Hannah wouldn't be returning to class for the rest of this year---and maybe never---and there were going to be many other things we would need help with besides Caitlin's immediate needs.

Since we didn't have a lot of information at this point, Mike wanted to wait. I felt that the sooner we let people know, the less the burden would be. It was a strange dynamic between us, dictated by our very different styles, but we compromised by narrowing the list down to a few essential people. What happened, of course, was by the beginning of the next week, so many people were involved we didn't have to ask for much, and if we did, there was a line of people waiting to do whatever we needed. We were so lucky to being living in such a caring community.

We sat side by side dealing with the mechanics of what had to happen and hadn't gotten to the real emotions we were going through. The silence that had settled over us was interrupted by one of the nurses coming in to tell us the biopsy was done. We both bounded up and out the door in a rush to the elevator. Our footsteps echoed as we crossed to the far side of the otherwise empty recovery room. Hannah's stretcher stood alone at the end of the huge room, a single nurse and Dr. Schwenn watching over her. My heart caught in my throat at the sight. Dr. Schwenn assured us all had gone well. I whispered a grateful prayer, my demons at bay for the moment.

The anesthesiologist had been correct in his prediction. She woke up chuckling about his joke. We kept talking with her as she slowly came out of the anesthesia. Dr. Schwenn stayed with us briefly and asked us more about our background and Hannah in particular. We both had taken an enormous liking to this very competent oncologist, and our trust continued to build. She told Hannah she would see her later upstairs, as she excused herself to work on finding out exactly which type of leukemia Hannah had.

We didn't know it at the time, but by getting the OR team there so quickly and having the biopsy done by noon, Dr. Schwenn was able to get samples on the two o'clock FedEx plane out of the Portland Jet Port to Dana Farber, the Mayo Clinic, and St. Jude's to have other specialists look at them. MCCP was part of an international consortium working to advance the care and treatment of children with cancer. She also called in a pathologist from the medical school to work with her the next day.

Although Hannah was recovered enough to go to her room, she was still very sleepy, wanted to rest, and wasn't particularly interested in food. We called Caitlin to see how she was doing and let her know the biopsy was done and Hannah was okay. We told her we would have Hannah call when she awoke. She was relieved, and told us she was glad she didn't try to go to the swim meet since she couldn't have concentrated on swimming. Being shy and very private, she didn't want to have to explain to anyone why she was upset.

Once Hannah was fully awake and had eaten something, I decided to take a short walk outside on the Western Promenade. The residential area next to the hospital was filled with beautiful old homes. I wondered if the people who lived in them were used to seeing people walking along the sidewalks with red eyes and runny noses from crying. My walk was short; because I was uncomfortable about walking around crying and fearful something might go wrong while I was away.

I reentered by one of the back doors in the oldest part of the hospital. The corridor led to the main entrance, but was lined by administrative offices, medical records, and other services. As I followed the signs to the lobby, one in particular caught my eye: CHAPEL. I hesitated for a moment, torn between wanting to get back to Hannah and my need for just such a sanctuary. I peered in. It was empty. I walked slowly to the front, sat down and gazed at the simple wooden altar above which was a beautiful lighted stained-glass window depicting the ocean, the hills, and a road leading to a lighthouse with a shining beacon. I worried, as I felt my tears start again, that I might never be able to sit alone without sobbing uncontrollably.

Taking the hymnal from the rack in front of me, I opened it randomly and saw the familiar words of "Abide with Me." Knowing I needed to find strength for this trial, I closed my eyes, took several deep, cleansing breaths, and let the familiar words of the hymn flow through my mind. Slowly I felt an inner calm spreading through me. This would be part of the way I survived. My tears stopped and I felt able to face the rest of the day.

I'd found a haven, and although I didn't stay long this first time, I knew where it was. I would use this and my daily meditation to cope emotionally. The clinical part of me would deal with what happened medically. I would use every bit of my knowledge and skills to get Hannah through this with the least amount of damage. I had cared for many very ill people in my career and given them the best I had to offer. I knew I would, by sheer force of will, if necessary, help her survive. If she died it wouldn't be for lack of trying on my part.

Around Hannah, I would be positive about the outcome, supporting her strength and helping her maintain a belief in her ability to beat the cancer. The core of me that was grieving, scared, and emotional would have to wait for places and times like this to be in the forefront. Only then would I allow myself to be vulnerable and needy.

Hannah was feeling better since she had eaten and was once again ensconced in her bed. She and Mike were settled in for the night and I was reassured by how much better she seemed. Now I wanted to be home for Caitlin. I trudged through the halls toward the front entrance of the hospital, my head down, thinking about the events of the last twenty-four hours. Once outside, I glanced up before crossing the street. On the other side, four or five teenagers stood smoking cigarettes. I froze and stared at them. My head felt as if it would explode with rage.

I fought the urge to beat them about the head and face while berating them for their stupidity. How could they be poisoning themselves and inviting cancer into their lives? My daughter was an athlete, had eaten healthy, and never even been exposed to smoking, but for some inexplicable reason had been stricken with cancer. It wasn't fair! I glared at them as I walked to the car. I had never felt such outrage over someone else's choice of lifestyle. How could they be so dumb? I fumed about it for the first part of my drive and then relegated it to the pile of "things I can do nothing about at the moment."

After an all-too-short evening with Caitlin and an only slightly better night's sleep, I was on my way back to the hospital through lighter Sunday morning traffic. When I arrived and saw Hannah, I felt my spirits sag. The previous night she had looked a little better, but now she was again pale, listless, and content to lie in bed with a book. They had started her on an antibiotic and had given her another blood transfusion, but she was visibly getting steadily worse.

Mike had slept better and was happy he'd had another night with her. He was, however, concerned about his soccer team. He knew many of them were worried about Hannah. Since there were no plans for any procedures or any other workup today, we both decided it would be good for him to go to the tournament and take news to the team.

After Mike left, I helped Hannah with her morning care. Once she was in a clean bed and we had time alone, I decided to talk with her about any questions she might have. I still felt guilty about not being able to talk with her about her diagnosis on Friday, and needed to know if there were other things she didn't understand.

"Are you worried about anything right now? Do you have any specific questions?"

She shook her head and said, "Not really. But do I have to keep the IV all the time?"

"Yep, you'll need to have one for the medicines like the antibiotics and the blood transfusions. Kinda stinks, huh?" I said.

She nodded.

"It must seem so weird having all of this happen so fast."

"Yeah, but I feel better as long as I can be in bed."

I sat down on her bed, pulled her into my arms.

"Oh, sweetie, this must be so hard. I don't know why God gave this to you. I don't know what's going to be happening in the next few days, but we'll do whatever it takes to get you through this. We'll do it together. We all love you so much, and if we could take this away, we would. I'm so sorry."

She rested her head on my shoulder and sighed.

"I don't know the reason this is happening, but I have to believe there is a purpose. This is all going to become a part of who you are. You're a very special girl and I know in my heart that you have an important purpose in life. I don't know yet what it is, but I have to believe this'll be a part of it."

She hugged me tighter and nodded as I said, "We will get through this together and do whatever has to be done, but I need something from you."

"What?" she mumbled into my shoulder.

"You need to believe that we can get rid of the cancer. Your job is to believe you will be able to get well, and our job with the medical staff is to do all that can be done to make it happen. I promise you that you will never be alone and we'll be there for you."

She pulled back from my shoulder and looked deeply into my eyes deciding if what I was saying was what I believed.

In her most serious voice, she said, "I can do that, Mom."

We sat for a long time snuggled up together. I wanted to believe we could survive this and she would become who she was meant to be in the process. I didn't really know if she could survive, but if I had any say in it, she would. She was a strong and courageous girl, and we would fight beside her no matter what we had to do. I wasn't certain what horrible events might await us in the next few days, but I could fight for Hannah to live for as long as it took!

She fell asleep and I took a break in the solarium. I carried all of the cancer-related informational books, pamphlets, and instructional materials we had been given with me. The large loose-leaf notebook from

Maine Children's Cancer Program had information about the treatment process, the issues we might face, and what hospitalization could be like for a child. Many of the side effects of treatment were similar to things I had known in caring for adult cancer patients. They could leave permanent damage and long-term disability; too disheartening to think about now.

I turned to the section on chemotherapy. There were pictures of smiling, bald-headed children with puffy faces. I wondered what their parents thought and if they would have recognized them if they hadn't been with them to see it happening. Having cared for mentally and physically handicapped kids, I knew that one forgot about their appearance and saw them as people, but I didn't know how I would feel about it with my own child.

As I read on about possible learning disabilities, damage to brain, heart, and other parts of the body, I cringed at the thought of those things happening to Hannah. What if she came out of this damaged or a totally different person? Would I trade her survival even if she weren't the same person? Who could make such a decision? Of course, at the rate she was going downhill, we didn't have any guarantee that she would even survive the next few days. What good did it do to even think about anything long term? Still, no matter how ill she looked, I was able to see her as my funny, athletic eleven-year-old, playing soccer, dancing, telling funny stories, and just being a fifth grader. I wondered how long that would last.

I put my head down on the back of the couch and thought about the last couple of days. I was stuck on just the word cancer, not having even thought through treatment. Were there any other choices? Could we *not* give her these poisons and still kill the cancer? I realized I was so scared I hadn't thought about anything but whatever they could do here or at some other treatment center. I just wanted Hannah to survive. Right now though, I didn't really know what I could do other than what was being done, so I gave up on reading the rest of the manual.

Just as I was about to go back to Hannah's room, our social worker, Liz, came into the solarium and sat beside me.

"How are you doing?" she asked.

"I don't really know. I think I'm still in shock."

"I'm sure you are. Have you had a chance to look through the materials about the program, and do you have any specific questions?"

I thought for a while before I said to her, "I'm sure you're a very nice person and a good social worker, but I don't want my child to *be* one of these children. I don't want her here. I don't want her to be sick!"

"I know this is hard. It isn't easy for any parent, but for you it must be a real role reversal. You don't really have any control being the parent and not the health care provider. I'm sure it must be very hard seeing her so sick and not being able to do anything. But there will be questions and issues that you need help with. Please let us give you support and help with whatever you need," she said.

"Thanks, but right now, I feel as if I need to just do what has to be done. If I admit how this feels, I'll probably end up a helpless puddle on the floor."

"I understand," she said.

Liz gave me a hug and then we walked back to Hannah's room together.

Her job wasn't an easy one. I appreciated the patience and support she offered and recognized that I needed it, but for now, my only way of coping with this without falling apart was to do the medical part by looking at it through professionally, not personally, tinted glasses. Back in Hannah's room, I put the large notebook entitled *A Journey of Hope* on the windowsill. I knew why they had given it that title, but at this moment, optimism and successful treatment outcomes weren't even on my radar.

Since Mike would be closer to home when he left the soccer tournament, we decided it made more sense for me to stay with Hannah. He would sleep at home and bring Caitlin so we could all be together for Memorial Day. It was the first of many nights I would spend on the only partially comfortable couch/bed in Hannah's hospital room.

When Mike and Caitlin arrived the next morning, Hannah cheered up immediately. Mike told her about the tournament and brought her cards from the team, which we put up in her room. He also demonstrated the "Hannah cheer" the team had done before each game. They had outplayed Mike's expectations for them in a very competitive tournament, falling just short of making the final day's playoffs. He felt that it had been a good thing that he had gone, since the players and families were all really worried about Hannah. She was sad that she couldn't play, but happy that the team did so well and proud that they did a cheer for her.

Dr. Schwenn had results from the bone marrow aspiration and biopsy. While Hannah and Caitlin watched a movie in her room, Mike and I went into the teen room with Dr. Schwenn to talk. Mike had spent the previous evening at home trolling the Internet researching the different types of leukemia. The results he found were not very encouraging.

Talking with Dr. Schwenn would give him a chance to understand the mechanisms of blood cell production and what had gone wrong to cause the leukemia.

"Your bone marrow makes red blood cells (RBCs), white blood cells (WBCs) and platelets (PLTs). The RBCs carry oxygen to all the cells in your body. If you don't have enough, you become anemic. If you don't have effective WBCs, you can't fight infections and you need platelets for your blood to clot," she said.

"Most of the symptoms we see are based on those problems. If the body can't fight infection, you get fevers and chills, and cuts or sores won't heal. Not having enough red blood cells makes you pale and really tired. It can also cause headaches. Without enough platelets, you bruise easily, get nosebleeds, or your gums bleed when you brush your teeth," she continued.

"Hannah didn't really have any bruising, and other than the ear infection, hasn't gotten any other infections. Does that mean her cancer isn't that bad?" I asked.

"We haven't quite determined her level. The amount of abnormal cells is rather low, so we initially didn't think this was acute myeloid leukemia, but with the testing from the biopsy and aspiration, it most likely is."

"I read about the various types of leukemia, but still don't get exactly what all that means," Mike said.

"I know this may sound complicated, but I'll try to make sense of it. There are four main types of leukemia with many subtypes. It's generally classified as either acute or chronic. In an acute type the abnormal cells are unable to mature properly. Those cells are called blasts and they continually reproduce and accumulate in the blood. Without treatment most patients with acute leukemia live only a few months. With chronic leukemia the cells partially mature, but not completely. They're not really normal and don't fight infection as well as normal cells. They also survive longer than normal cells and can crowd out the other healthy blood cells."

"So Hannah has the acute type of leukemia?" Mike asked.

"It looks that way. We also classify according to the type of white blood cell affected. If the cancer affects lymphocytes, it's classified as lymphocytic leukemia. If the granulocytes or monocytes are involved, then it is called myeloid leukemia. Each of the types, lymphocytic and myeloid, are divided up as acute or chronic so we call them acute lymphocytic leukemia (ALL), chronic lymphocytic leukemia (CLL), acute myeloid leukemia (AML), and chronic myeloid leukemia (CML)," Dr. Schwenn said.

"Which of these is worse, or is one as bad as another?" Mike asked.

"We don't like any of them. I thought yesterday that because Hannah is so ill, but doesn't have a lot of circulating blast cells [immature white cells], that she might have chronic myeloid leukemia. Kids don't do so well with that one, which we usually see in adults. Unless you can have a bone marrow transplant, it has a poor outcome."

"But you don't think that is what she has, right?" Mike asked.

"We'll know more once we've heard back from the pathologists at the various centers where I sent Hannah's slides from the bone marrow aspiration and biopsy. But you're right, it doesn't seem to be CML," she said.

Dr. Schwenn went on to explain the importance of being able to start chemotherapy quickly, even if they didn't have all of the genetic markers identified. This meant Hannah would need a central intravenous line surgically placed in her chest.

"I managed to have Hannah added to the surgical schedule tomorrow. We'll put in the central line, look inside her chest cavity to see what is causing the shadow around her lungs that we saw on the CT, and do a spinal tap to make certain she doesn't have any cancer cells in her spinal fluid."

"Do you know what time she'll have surgery tomorrow?" I asked.

"No. She's an add-on, so it will depend on how long all the other surgeries take, but it will definitely be after lunchtime."

While Mike and Dr. Schwenn continued to discuss what he had read about AML and CML for which there was a new drug that seemed promising, I tuned out and thought back over the last four days. Before we had a diagnosis, time dragged by, but now everything was happening at hyper-speed. I wondered how families and patients with no medical background coped with this kind of overload. Even though I had a high level of medical knowledge, I could barely take it all in. I didn't know if it was better to be ignorant of all that could go wrong or if it was good to be able to anticipate possible complications. Actually, I didn't want to face either.

I was pulled out of my reflections by Dr. Schwenn asking, "How do you want us to talk with Hannah about what we will be doing tomorrow?"

"You need to be really direct with her. She won't trust what you say if she senses that she isn't being given the full story. She is very, very intelligent and will understand most everything you need to tell her. I think it will help if she knows what's happening," I said.

"I'd like to talk to her now, if that's okay," Dr. Schwenn said.

Mike and I returned to Hannah's room and told her that Dr. Schwenn wanted to come in to explain what would be happening in the next few days. Caitlin, Mike, and I sat together on the couch as Dr. Schwenn came in with books and reports and sat down next to the bed.

"Hannah, this is our time to talk and have your questions answered. Your parents and your sister can be here, but they can't ask questions or talk. Is that okay?"

Hannah looked at us and then back at Dr. Schwenn and nodded.

Dr. Schwenn opened a medical textbook to the section on leukemia and explained, "Leukemia occurs when one abnormal white blood cell is broken and begins to clone itself over and over. These cells don't mature or function properly and they don't die when they should. They aren't as able to fight infection as normal white blood cells are. As they continue to build up in the bloodstream, other healthy blood cells are crowded out. If the bone marrow isn't able to produce these other cells, anemia, bruising, and frequent infections can happen. The bone marrow isn't able to produce new bone and things like fibrous dysplasia can occur, such as in your jaw. The bone marrow wasn't able to produce healthy bone and that caused the area without bone they saw on your X-ray at the orthodontist's office. The piece that flaked off was fibrous tissue that hadn't become bone."

Hannah looked at the pictures of blood cells and nodded.

"Hannah, your spleen is so swollen because one of its main jobs is to filter out and destroy old blood cells. Because there are so many abnormal ones, it can't keep up with the overload," she continued.

"Does that make my stomach hurt?" Hannah asked.

"I think that's part of it. Your spleen is also so big that your stomach is getting squished. That's why you don't feel like eating, and when you do, you feel full right away."

"Oh," Hannah said and glanced over at us and nodded.

"The other part of this problem is that, for some reason, your body doesn't recognize the broken cells and kill them. Your immune system is supposed to recognize cells that are different and get rid of them. Most cells also have a specific life span, and when they have functioned as mature cells for the right amount of time, they die. The problem in leukemia is that both of these problems are happening. Your body doesn't recognize the abnormal cells and they continue to clone themselves, stay in an immature state, and then crowd out your healthy cells," Dr. Schwenn said.

Hannah glanced at us from time to time for confirmation, but listened intently. She asked questions as Dr. Schwenn told her about the need for a central IV line and how it would work. She explained about getting transfusions while she was being treated, and that they would give her medicine to keep her from feeling sick when she received the chemotherapy. It was a very reassuring talk. I didn't know whether it had answered all of Hannah's questions, but now we had more information about the plans for care.

All too soon, it was time for Mike and Caitlin to leave. It was hard to hold back the tears, knowing that I wouldn't see them for at least a couple of days and we had no idea what might happen to Hannah with the surgery. They both held Hannah and told her how much they loved her, and reassured her that we would all talk on the phone.

I hugged Caitlin tightly. "Remember your only job right now is to continue with school and do well on your exams. If you still don't want to tell anyone at Berwick what has happened, that's okay, but I have spoken with your teachers and advisor so they're available for help and support. And of course, call me any time just to talk. I'll call every day before you go to school and when you get home. Okay?"

She nodded and clung to me for just an instant and then they left.

Hannah snuggled down in bed and watched TV while I sat on the couch reading until Dr. Schwenn returned with the pediatric surgeons who wanted to examine Hannah before her surgery tomorrow. Hannah liked the chief surgeon, and was especially impressed by his lab coat, which had a picture of Big Bird covering the back of it. He discussed what they would be doing, and I signed the consent form for the surgery.

I helped Hannah get cleaned up and then converted the couch into a bed for myself. I felt so tired that I thought I would fall asleep immediately, but everything bothered me. Even with the curtain drawn and the door closed, there was still too much light and noise. As nurses came in and out all night, I heard every beep of any of the machinery, including the IV pump, electronic blood-pressure cuff, and thermometer. The window into the hall and the one over my bed both had blinds, but a lot of light spilled in around them. I knew I was blaming the conditions for not being able to shut my mind off, but finally I resigned myself to the reality that deep, restful sleep was probably out of the question for the foreseeable future. Instead I began visualization and relaxation exercises in hopes that at least reducing my stress level would help me face the trials of tomorrow.

Chapter 8

HOOKED UP

Central Line Insertion: surgical placement, under general anesthesia, of an intravenous catheter into a large vessel such as the vena cava to provide a long-term IV port for the administration of chemotherapy, transfusions, or medications.

Hannah and I both awoke early the next morning. It would have been nice to sleep in, but the general noise level, the amount of light in our room, and the surgical team rounds didn't allow that. Once they left, I helped her to the bathroom to wash up. I stood at the sink filling a basin with warm water and glanced back just as her face went white and she started to fall. I grabbed her and pushed her head down toward her knees while guiding her to the commode to sit down.

"I'm going to be sick, Mom!"

Still holding onto her, I dumped the basin in the sink and put it on the floor in front of her. I grabbed a wash cloth, ran cold water on it, and placed it on the back of her neck.

After a few minutes, she said, "I'm a little better; can I just go back to my bed?"

I carried her to the bed. Trying not to show my worry about her increasing weakness, I told her I would treat her to a bed bath and tried to make a joke out of it. She was too tired to do much but smile a little.

I let her rest until she felt better and then did a quick bed bath, helped her brush her teeth, and braided her hair. Even with my doing most everything, she needed to sleep when we were done.

While she rested from her morning care, her nurse started a unit of platelets and gave her some medication to improve clotting during surgery. Amazingly, she woke up an hour or so later, announced she was hungry, and made a joke about the blood transfusion giving her an appetite. We laughed because now she couldn't eat until after surgery. Just our luck! This incredible child still had her sense of humor even though she clearly felt much worse today than yesterday. I swallowed my tears and sat with her watching a movie, pretending this was going to be okay.

Even though she didn't like going back to surgery, she said she was fine with getting a central line. It meant that she wouldn't have to have blood drawn from veins in her hands and arms, plus multiple medications could be given without additional IVs. It also meant she could wear regular clothes, since it would exit on her chest wall instead of from one of her arms. I wasn't sure she really understood what it would mean to have tubes coming out of her chest for the next few months. I wasn't certain I did either.

While Hannah was under anesthesia, the surgeon planned to do a thoracoscopy (make a hole her chest wall) to examine the area around her right lung. He would use an endoscope, a narrow tube with a mirror or camera attached to it, to do the exam. This technique would let them examine the area without making a large incision. Hopefully, this would mean less chance for postoperative complications, as the small incision would heal more quickly and be less painful.

The final procedure under anesthesia would be a spinal tap to examine her spinal fluid looking for cancer cells that might have crossed the blood/brain barrier. If they had, it would not be a good sign, since having cancer in her brain could mean many neurological complications. To help prevent this, they planned to replace the amount of spinal fluid they removed for testing with a dose of ARA-C, a chemotherapy drug. The possibility that, if she survived, she might have long-term physical disabilities and be mentally impaired made me shudder. I had to immediately put the image out of my mind. I didn't have the energy to worry about that now; I would face it if and when I had to.

Hannah fell asleep again and I sat on the couch staring out the window. I felt as if this were a constant lesson in living in the *now*. I was normally an *anticipator*. I tried to think ahead about what could happen and then prevent any problems. It was probably a skill that made me a very good nurse, but it also carried over into my personal life. Despite years of yoga and meditation practice, I didn't live in the here and now. These last few days had done more toward teaching me to be present in the now than all of my previous meditation efforts. I was being forced to learn this because my energy was limited. Wasting it worrying about what future terrors awaited us would drain me completely.

My resolve to be in the now didn't, however, stop the medical part of my brain from thinking about all of the possible complications and what they might find during surgery. I hoped whatever was causing her pain and shortness of breath wasn't more bad news. The droop on the left side of her face was more pronounced this morning, but she didn't have the pain in her back. Still, we needed to know the cause. We had made it this far, but our episode in the bathroom was proof she was getting weaker. This moment was all we had. She was still alive and they were doing what needed to be done to give her a chance at survival, but there were no promises of a good outcome. My worst fear was that she wouldn't even survive long enough to start chemotherapy.

I needed to hear Mike's voice, even if it was just at the other end of the phone. We were both really scared, but knew there wasn't anything else we could do right now. I told him what the day's schedule was and we agreed I would call at each stage. I hated doing this long distance, but that was our reality.

Shortly before noon, the anesthesiologist examined Hannah while I signed the anesthesia consent form. They could come to take her to the OR any time now. Outwardly I was calm and matter-of-fact about what would happen in the OR, but inside I wanted to have a tantrum and give in to my panic. This side of the bed certainly wasn't fun.

Although I would like to believe that I had provided supportive, quality nursing care innumerable times for patients and families going through preoperative experiences, I now realized nothing prepared anyone for the intensity of the fear involved in sending a child to surgery, especially with the word cancer in the diagnosis. I had assured families that their loved one would do well and we would provide them with excellent care.

What had I been talking about? Placing your child in someone else's hands was an act of faith. How could we, in the patient care field, be so glib with our assurances about how any medical intervention would play out? My insides felt as if they were being hit with jolts of liquid fear. It physically hurt to be this afraid. I knew I would never again talk with any patient or family member without this awareness coloring my interactions.

Shortly after noon, an orderly arrived with the OR stretcher. With all of the last-minute preoperative checks completed, we were on our way. At the entrance to the holding area, we were both issued OR caps to cover our hair, and I put nonconductive booties over my shoes. I sat beside Hannah's bed in a rocking chair as she rested and snuggled Lovey Bear. Hand-holding was our communication and security blanket for now.

I was grateful that when our turn finally came, they allowed me to go all the way to the OR suite with her. I walked beside the stretcher holding tightly to her hand. When the nurse opened the door, I shivered as the cold air rushed out. The door was too narrow for us all to squeeze through, so I had to let go of her hand, but I stopped them. I hugged her to me and gave her a kiss. She smiled and handed me Lovey.

"I love you, big bug. Lovey and I will be waiting for you when you wake up."

"I love you, too, Mom."

The nurses wheeled her to the middle of the room to the narrow metal OR table, where three huge, bright lights made it center stage. They transferred her onto the table as I stood so she could see me smiling encouragement. Her smile wavered a little as they draped her. Suddenly, as they began injecting the anesthetic into her IV, she winced and began to writhe and cry in pain. Before I could shout at them to stop hurting her, she was asleep. The circulating nurse closed the door. I stood alone in the corridor dripping tears on Lovey.

I called Mike, but didn't tell him about the IV being inflamed or about her pain as she went under anesthesia. It was enough that *I* was upset; he didn't need to be any more worried than he already was.

With the surgery scheduled to take about an hour, the nurses in pre-op had suggested I go to the cafeteria to eat. They would know to find me either there or in Hannah's room if they needed me. After twenty minutes of putting good food, which turned to cardboard, into my mouth, I gave up and went back to her room to wait. I stared out the window, tried to read my book, and watched the slow movement of the hands on the large clock above the door. Tired from lack of sleep, and not knowing how much opportunity I would have to rest in the next twenty-four hours, I lay down. I must have dozed off because I awoke with a jolt to someone saying my name. Guiltily, I bolted upright and tried to clear my head of sleep.

One of the pediatric surgeons was standing beside me. He said, "Hannah will be going into the recovery area in a few minutes. You can go down there and sit with her while she wakes up."

"How did she do? What did you find?" I asked.

"First of all, the placement of the Broviac catheter [central venous IV line] went well. We put it on the right side of her chest. The really good news is that her spinal fluid was clear of any cancer and we gave her a dose of ARA-C. We also took 600 milliliters [about 2 ½ cups] of fluid from around her right lung. Luckily, we were able to do this through the scope, so she doesn't need a chest tube to keep her right lung inflated."

"That's a relief! Did you find the cause of her back pain and shortness of breath?" I asked.

"We think that the pain was caused by the fluid, but the fluid was there because of what are called chloromas [pearly green, sterile pus sacs] in the space between her lung and the lining of her chest. We removed them and took multiple biopsies."

"I've never heard of chloromas. What causes them?"

"We think they may be related to all of the circulating blast cells forming clusters. The pressure that they and the fluid around her lung caused was most likely the source of her pain. The droop on the left side of her face was also probably from the pressure the fluid was causing. It shifted her lungs a little toward the left side and put pressure on some nerves. Her lung could still collapse, so she will need a lot of encouragement to cough and deep breathe to prevent that and a post-op pneumonia."

"Thank you. It's good to know why she was having the back pain, and I'm really relieved that there wasn't any cancer in the spinal fluid."

I couldn't think of anything else to ask, plus I really wanted to run past him to get to the recovery room as quickly as possible. I thanked him and speed-walked to the elevators. As I rode to the basement, I thought about what he had told me. There was definitely some good news, but it was dwarfed by the bigger issues of treating her cancer. His tone hadn't been negative about her chances, but he also hadn't sounded particularly upbeat and optimistic either.

For the third time in three days, I walked through the two sets of double doors into the recovery room. Today, I hardly recognized it as the same place. Hannah wasn't the only patient now. The rows of postoperative beds, separated by sliding track curtains hanging from the ceiling, were all full. The quiet of Saturday was gone, replaced by a cacophony of sounds: beeping cardiac monitors, IV pump alarms, ringing phones, and nurses encouraging patients to cough or turn. The smells of anesthesia, surgical tape, and a particular human odor I associated with distress and fear hung in the air.

Postoperative care required individual monitoring for each patient. At the open end of each curtained cubicle was a mini mobile nurse's station complete with medications and emergency supplies where the nurse assigned to that patient recorded vital signs and patient status every fifteen minutes or less.

The charge nurse indicated Hannah was in cubicle 5 down on the left side of the room. I could see the curtain with cartoon characters ahead as I counted cubicles. I stood at the opening and looked at Hannah lying small and fragile on the large bed. There were traces of tears on her cheeks. Her nurse turned from checking the vital signs monitors and motioned me to come in. I introduced myself to her, then put down the bed rail, leaned over Hannah and kissed her forehead.

"She's been uncomfortable and upset because she wants a drink of water, but I don't think she has a lot of pain because she has the PCA pump [continuous low-dose morphine infusion system]. It's that her throat and mouth are dry from being intubated during surgery, but she can only have ice chips."

"I'm sorry she's upset. I'm sure she doesn't really understand why she can't have water. Is she waking up more than just when you take vital signs and turn her?" I asked.

"No. She only cries when I wake her. You can sit here with her until she wakes up enough to go upstairs."

"Thanks." I took Hannah's hand and kissed her face again, saying, "Hi, sweet girl. You're just fine. The surgery is over and Mom and Lovey are here again."

She opened her eyes a tiny slit, reached for Lovey and croaked, "Mommy, my throat hurts and I'm thirsty."

"I know, but you can only have some ice chips for now until you're really awake. They don't want you to get sick and throw up from having too much in your stomach. Can you do that, buggy?"

She nodded as I spooned a few ice chips into her mouth. She fell asleep again and I sat down in the rocking chair beside the stretcher and held her hand. She had come through the surgery, her vital signs were normal, and she didn't have any bleeding. At least we had gotten this far without a disaster. Sore throat and ice chip issues I could live with.

At the next fifteen-minute vital sign check, the nurse asked, "Do you want to see her dressings and the central line?"

"Sure."

The two small dressings on the right side of her back where they had made the incisions to look inside her chest had no signs of bleeding on the gauze pads. The nurse turned her onto her back and unsnapped her gown to show me the central line. I swallowed hard as I looked through the transparent sterile dressing which covered the right center of her thin chest. I knew what central lines looked like; they were on some really ill patient's chest, not on my daughter's. I turned away and took another deep breath.

A gauze dressing covered the site of the line's insertion into the subclavian vein just under her collarbone, but I could see the faint outline of the tunnel they had created under her skin to bring the tubing down to the center of her chest. There was a bulge under her skin at the opening where the central line came out to the surface; it was the cuff around which, in time, her skin would grow to help hold the line in place and seal it against outside organisms. Where it exited the skin on her chest, there were fresh sutures and a 2 x 2 gauze pad. The part of the central line that forked at a Y joint was visible under the see-through dressing material. Below the dressing on her upper abdomen lay the two ports with their special adaptors hooked up to the intravenous tubing that was giving her pain medication and IV solutions.

The clinical aspects of the dressings and catheter didn't bother me; I'd seen them many times before. But they looked different on Hannah's chest; we owned them. Caring for them wasn't just a clinical task, it was crucial to preventing an infection that could kill her. I wondered what she would think, when she finally came fully awake and saw, felt, and had to live with this new attachment to her body. I bit my lip and stroked her cheek. *This better be leading to an increased chance of survival,* I thought.

As each vital signs check passed, Hannah became more and more alert, but was no less unhappy about not being able to drink water. The anesthesiologist came by to see her, as did one of the pediatric surgical residents. They both assured me she was doing great and had come through the surgery quite well. For some strange reason, I felt proud of the fact that she had done so well and grateful that we seemed to have been somewhat lucky so far in what they had found.

Toward evening, she was recovered enough to be moved back to her room. I had talked to both Mike and Caitlin to tell them how Hannah was doing, and they were both relieved. I held the phone to Hannah's ear so they could both tell her they loved her, but she didn't have the energy to talk.

Her room no longer looked like a place to hang out and watch movies. Computerized monitoring equipment kept track of all her vital functions, provided IV solutions, and kept her pain under control. They needed to keep her right lung from collapsing, check for bleeding, and monitor her for any signs of impending infection. Every half hour, she needed to be turned, and made to take deep breaths, and cough. She didn't like me or the nurses pushing her to do these things, but I explained to her they were really important if she was going to get better. I knew how close to the edge we were if we weren't aggressive in her postoperative care. She was weak from the cancer, which made her that much more vulnerable to infection and other complications.

She hated being awakened because she could still have only a few ice chips and tiny sips of water so she didn't vomit. She also wanted the annoying duck-bill shaped clamp on her index finger removed. It measured the amount of oxygen in her blood (O2 saturation), which was essential to knowing how her lungs were doing. The oxygen tubing prongs in her nose were another petty annoyance, but also essential.

If I never again used my nursing skills for anything other than this, they would have been the most valuable thing I possessed. As I helped her turn, got her to take deep breaths, and fed her ice chips, I thought back on all of the postoperative patients for whom I had provided care over the years. I had assisted them to do all of these same uncomfortable but crucial procedures to assure their best chance of recovery, but this felt very different. I couldn't divorce myself from her pain and tears. The urgency I felt about being on top of any changes in her physical state was intense. I made no attempt to be involved with any of the equipment. The very competent nurses who were caring for her could do all of that, but I used all of my nursing knowledge to be her advocate and give her the best care I could.

At some point, I realized it had gotten dark outside. I made up the couch into my bed, checked in with Mike and Caitlin to give them an update, and tried to rest for a while.

I had just fallen into a deep sleep when the alarms on the O2 saturation monitor went off. I jumped up to check on Hannah as two nurses came running in.

"Hannah, you need to take some deep breaths!" one of the nurses said.

I helped Hannah sit up a little higher in her bed as she coughed and took a couple of deep breaths.

"Her O2 sats are dropping every time she falls into deep sleep. We like to keep them above 92 to 94%, but hers keep dropping down into the 70s. Don't worry; the monitor lets us know any time they drop lower, so we can get her to breathe deeply and cough," Tracey, her nurse, assured me.

I hugged Hannah and held her until she fell asleep again. Watching the monitor for a while before lying down myself, I felt reassured, but not for long. The whole scenario played itself out again a few minutes later. I felt like a jack-in-the-box popping up from my bed every time the alarms sounded.

When the night nurse took her vital signs around eleven o'clock, Hannah's temperature was 104.4F. Several nurses came in, drew blood cultures, hung another IV with an antibiotic in it, and checked her lungs and dressings. Concerned this might be the beginning of a postoperative pneumonia, they pushed her even harder with the coughing and deep breathing. I hovered, gave Hannah verbal encouragement, and tried not to give in to my own fears.

Somewhere around 2:00 in the morning, I woke up when Hannah began to cry as Tracey asked her to take deep breaths.

I got up to help turn Hannah and comfort her.

"I am so sorry you're upset, sweetie, but crying is also a really good way to take deep breaths and is probably good for you right now."

"That's not a very nice thing to say, Mom. Crying is okay?"

"I know it sounds mean, but if it helps your lung to stay inflated and improves your oxygen saturation, I'm okay with it. I'm not trying to be mean. You know I love you and wouldn't do anything that hurts unless it's absolutely necessary."

"I know," she said with a sigh.

She dutifully took her deep breaths and coughed. I held her until she stopped crying and fell back to sleep. The alarms didn't immediately go off again, so I took a moment to walk outside into the hall. Tracey was at the nurse's station and as I approached, she said, "We think you're a really good nurse. We took a vote and decided to hire you, so we ordered some nursing scrubs."

I laughed. "Thank you, but the only job I can handle right now is being a full-time mom. Anyway, I hated working in pediatrics with sick kids. It always made me feel so sad."

From their comments, I realized that, to all outward appearances, I must look as if I were handling all this stress quite well. But inside there were moments when my fear would sneak up on me and make me so jittery I felt as if my movements were being controlled by an uncoordinated puppet master. I had to try to figure out how to breathe again every time this happened.

Before going back into Hannah's room, I stretched and took a couple of deep breaths, and then realized that Dr. Schwenn was sitting at the desk.

Surprised, I asked, "What are you doing here so late?"

"Hannah's really ill. Where else would I be?"

Tears welled up in my eyes and my throat tightened as I breathed a prayer of gratitude that we had chosen this place. I allowed myself one little glimmer of hope. With this much help, maybe she would survive.

Chapter 9

THE BATTLE BEGINS

*Chemotherapy: the treatment of cancer with drugs
that kill abnormal cells as well as many normal cells.*

When Hannah stabilized around 4 A.M., I lay down again to rest. I must have fallen into a deeper sleep than I realized, because the sun in my face woke me and for a moment I couldn't remember where I was. When I did and it was quiet, I jumped out of bed and jerked the curtain aside. I blew out a breath, relieved to see Hannah sleeping and the alarms quiet. I sat back down on my bed shaking and remembering the same feeling of fear when the girls were babies and slept through a feeding for the first time. Now, for some reason, I had thought she hadn't made it and no one had woken me.

Relieved, I called Mike to tell him she was doing a bit better. He was reassured and grateful. Caitlin was doing okay and had made it to the bus for school with no trouble, and he was on his way to work. I told him I would call back after rounds.

Hannah woke up when the pediatric surgeons came in, examined her, and announced their satisfaction with her progress in recovering from the surgery. All of her dressings were clean, with no signs of bleeding or infection, and she didn't have a fever, thanks to the IV antibiotics. Her right lung was still inflated with no signs of postoperative pneumonia. Her only problems were diarrhea and stomach cramps.

Her nurse for the day, Disey, did an assessment of Hannah, checked the central line dressing site, the IV pump, and all of Hannah's surgical dressings before I started her morning care. They still needed to be aggressive about deep breathing and coughing, so the nurse brought an incentive spirometer (a device to help her take deep breaths and cough) for Hannah to use. Even after learning how, she didn't want to use it.

"It hurts in my shoulder and back when I cough and do all of that," she said.

"You need to push the plunger on the PCA pump if you're having pain and then do the coughing and deep breathing."

Her face crumpled and tears filled her eyes.

"I don't want to. It makes me feel bad."

"How does it make you feel bad?" I asked.

"I get cramps and feel like I'm going to toss."

Hannah was refusing the pain medication. I gave it some thought and was pretty certain the culprit might be the morphine which could cause those side effects.

I found Disey, and told her I thought Hannah might not be using the PCA pump to control her pain because the morphine was giving her diarrhea and cramps.

"Is there anything else she can have for pain?" I asked.

"Sure. Some kids don't do very well with the morphine. She has an order for acetaminophen. I'll let the resident know and we can switch her," Disey said.

Once Hannah was off the PCA pump, she started to feel a little better and we were able to finish up her bath and bed change. With the new pain medication, she was even willing to use the incentive spirometer.

After working the entire holiday weekend, Dr. Schwenn was not the covering oncologist today. We met another of the MCCP oncologists, Dr. Annie Rossi, who came in to explain about the plan to start the chemotherapy the next day. Treatment would begin based on what they knew now. They hoped to have the final genotype testing done, but they would begin with the same induction chemotherapy agents regardless of the exact genotype of AML.

Dr. Rossi asked to meet with Mike and me to discuss what they had learned so far and introduce us to the road map for Hannah's treatment. I called Mike back to tell him. They also wanted Caitlin to come so they could do HLA typing on all of us (Human leukocyte antigen-proteins or markers found on most human cells which your immune system uses to tell which cells are a part of you and which aren't.) If Hannah were able to get into remission with chemotherapy and if we were able to find a match, then a choice would be made as to whether she would continue to have chemotherapy or receive a bone marrow transplant (BMT).

The first place they would look for a match was within the immediate family, and in our case, that was Caitlin. The odds of Caitlin being a perfect match were around 30 to 35%. If she were not, then we would have to rely on the International Bone Marrow Registry. The first step would be a blood test to look for antigens on Caitlin's cells and tissues which might match with antigens on Hannah's cells and tissues. Since these antigens tell the body whether tissue is "other" or "self", they're used to determine a donor match for transplantation. Everyone inherits half of their antigens from the father and half from the mother. Unless you have an identical twin, your pattern is unique to you, but someone related by blood is more likely to have a similar pattern than a stranger would be. A close match is essential so the donated bone marrow won't be rejected.

Hannah's face lit up and she actually smiled when Mike and Caitlin walked in the door. It was good to see a smile on her face. I had one too, and it came from having us all together in the same place with Hannah still alive. After we caught up on all that had happened in the last two days, Mike, Caitlin, and I trooped down to the lab for the blood drawing. I knew Caitlin didn't like to have her blood drawn, but she was willing to do anything to help Hannah, and if we were lucky, there just might be a match.

After we returned, Hannah and Caitlin settled in to watch a video while Mike and I met with Dr. Rossi.

"We have the genetic typing results and if there can be any good news in this situation, we do have some," she said.

"This is acute myeloid leukemia of the type M2," she explained. "The subtype's important because different types of therapy may need to be used based on that. The M refers to myeloblasts, which are an unmatured type of white blood cell. Hannah's bone marrow smears showed she does have myeloblasts as the dominant type of abnormal cell. We analyzed these to look for a specific pattern of cells to determine which type is involved."

"Is that a good type?" Mike asked.

"There are eight M types. Each designation is based on finding certain types and patterns of cells in the patient's blood and bone marrow. Once we determine the type of abnormal cell, we use an international protocol to determine which chemotherapy drugs will be most effective."

Mike asked, "So what does this mean in Hannah's case, and is there any better outcome from one type versus another?"

"Hannah has a type associated with a more positive outcome. Leukemia, being a disorder of the bone marrow, occurs when one abnormal white blood cell, called a progenitor cell, begins to self-clone. The clones don't mature, don't fight infection well, and don't die at the rate normal white blood cells do. The initial source of the damage which caused the original abnormal cell to replicate frequently isn't known, and we also don't know why the cell is able to go on cloning."

"Why didn't Hannah's immune system destroy these cells, if they're abnormal?" I asked.

"For cancer to develop, the immune system has to fail to recognize the cloned cells as abnormal and not destroy them. What causes most of the symptoms is that the abnormal cells just keep reproducing and not dying off, thus crowding out the normal cells."

"You said you know the genotype as well," Mike said.

"Yes, we do. This is also some good news. The importance of the typing is related, not only the M2 type, but the chromosomal changes. That determines how treatable it is. The translocation of chromosomes 8 and 21 [t(8;21)] has a more favorable outcome, and this is what Hannah has."

"So, what does this really mean?" Mike asked.

"It means we have experience with this type of AML and the protocol we use has had some good outcomes," Dr. Rossi said.

Still not satisfied, Mike asked, "What are our chances with this type?"

"There is a 60 to 68% chance of a cure, and in England there have been reports of even better results, somewhere around 78%."

"Do you mean getting into remission or lifetime cure?" Mike asked.

"There is about an 80% remission rate and a 40 to 50% five-year relapse-free remission rate. When we reach that benchmark, it is considered a cure," she said.

Mike and I exchanged glances as I let out an audible sigh. Hannah had a chance. Mike squeezed my hand and relaxed back into his chair. We spent the rest of the meeting going over the treatment road map, which called for five rounds of chemotherapy. Each round would consist of an induction phase and, after a few days, a consolidation phase. The first round would be considered an induction to (we hoped) put her in remission. All of the additional rounds would be an effort to consolidate that gain. It seemed rather like shinnying up a rope with knots in it. After struggling to the next knot, you needed to hold there a bit, not sliding back, before you could make more progress. There were no firm dates for any of the other rounds, but the first one would start tomorrow and ten days later they would give the second part of the first round. The timing of the next rounds would depend on how well she responded and whether she developed complications that delayed treatment.

Our course was set and we were on the road whether we wanted to be or not. I couldn't think beyond just getting started with the treatment. All I had really heard from the whole meeting was that Hannah had a chance to survive. The statistics were in our favor if she didn't develop complications, and if she responded to the chemotherapy, and if...too many ifs. I could only think about now.

Preventing nausea during chemotherapy was important. Hannah would start those medications today and continue them around the clock during each phase of chemotherapy. Hopefully, this would keep her from feeling sick. The theory was that if she didn't learn to associate the chemotherapy with vomiting and feeling really ill, these symptoms would be less likely to occur. There had been some studies that had shown if kids associated getting chemotherapy with feeling sick, they actually started vomiting on the way to treatment just from the memory of feeling so sick. If we could prevent this happening, we definitely wanted to.

After phone calls to worried family and friends, we sat in Hannah's room laughing and talking. Before I was ready for them to leave, Mike and Caitlin left for home. Hannah wouldn't admit it while they were there, but she was tired out by being awake so long. I was tired too, but was afraid to sleep deeply. Instead, I slept when Hannah did and got up for every vital signs check.

Thursday morning Hannah felt better. She had slept more and transfusions of whole blood and platelets had also helped. She was still unable to get out of bed, but she ate a little breakfast and tolerated my giving her a full bed bath. I washed her hair while she was still lying in bed by using a basin and the tray table at the top of her bed. With her long hair combed and braided, she didn't have to worry about bed tangles. After her bath, she watched TV and played around with the spirometer. She proudly told me she had figured out a way to make it work without having to take such a deep breath. Her lungs were doing okay, but I gave her a hard time about cheating on the job. She agreed not to cheat, but secretly I took that as a very good sign. She felt well enough to be up to no good!

I was happy Hannah felt like eating something. She seemed to be taking this all in stride. I thought about how I would feel if I were in that bed, and I wondered if I would be able to handle all that had happened with such aplomb.

Before they started the first chemotherapy drug, Danorubicin, they needed to do an echocardiogram (a test which measures the health of the heart muscles and how efficiently they work) to see if her heart was okay. It would be important to document the condition of her heart before they started since the Danorubicin (an anti-tumor antibiotic) could damage heart muscle. A technician brought the machine into her room and explained how it worked. Because of her central line, Hannah's only concern was whether pressing on her chest would hurt. It didn't bother her that much, and she liked seeing the images of her beating heart on the computer screen. The technician explained what she was seeing and to my relief, the results showed she had a healthy athlete's heart.

Even though our conversation with Dr. Rossi had made me feel better about our chances and I was eager to start treatment, I hadn't really faced the reality of chemotherapy. While the echocardiogram was being done, I thought again about the potential for a permanent disability from the treatment. Everything seemed to be a tradeoff. If we didn't take these risks, she probably wouldn't survive. If we did and she ended up disabled, we would have to live with that. Perhaps we would be lucky.....

As much as I wanted treatment to start and thought I was ready for this next step, the sight of that first bag of bright red intravenous Danorubicin that Disey brought into the room brought me up short. This was real, she really did have cancer and she really was being treated with life-destroying anti-cancer drugs. Intellectually I knew she had cancer, but emotionally those thoughts had been on hold while I focused on her postoperative care. Watching the chemotherapy drug infuse into her body slammed the message home. It was too late to turn back now; we stepped into the void.

Until that moment, I had never understood why cancer patients and their families accepted the recommended treatment without question. The word cancer alone generated a whole world of meaning that couldn't be understood unless that word was applied to you or someone you loved. For so long, this diagnosis had been a death sentence, and despite tremendous improvements in the treatment options, it still engendered that same fear; a fear so paralyzing that a choice about treatment wasn't one.

At this point Hannah's survival depended on the chemotherapy killing the cancer cells and allowing her body to rebuild healthy bone marrow. Of course, in that process other healthy cells would also be destroyed, and the process of curing her could make her very ill and potentially even kill her. In my perfect world, no child would have such toxic drugs; but that world didn't exist anymore. Without immediate treatment, the person I loved beyond reason would die.

I wracked my brain for the possible sources of that first aberrant cell which had started the cancer. Was it the unusual flu she had in late December? Did that particular virus break some RNA in her white blood cells in its passage through her body? Was it something in the water or air where we lived? Could it be some chemical she had been exposed to in our neighborhood or someplace we had visited? Was Caitlin somehow at risk too, or had her immune system recognized the abnormal cells and killed them? All of these questions ate at me. We would probably never have a definitive answer, but in the meantime, my only hope was that this treatment would put Hannah into remission. So I sat quietly watching the red fluid flow into her central line, and consciously suspended negative thoughts about what it could do to her.

Chapter 10
BEHIND CLOSED DOORS

*Isolation: The process of separating somebody or something
from others, or the fact of being alone and apart from others.*

Hannah had been diagnosed a week ago. Today was her second day of chemotherapy, and she was becoming more stable with each passing day. When Mike arrived for the weekend, I would be able to go home. I had mixed feelings about leaving Hannah, but I knew I needed a break. Sleep deprivation had taken its toll, and I knew I wouldn't be any good to her if I didn't get some time to decompress.

While Hannah had been so critical, I'd had little time to think about anything else. Even so, I was still acutely aware of Caitlin's needs. I was looking forward to spending a couple of days with her. I missed her and felt sad about missing the last part of her freshman year of high school. Talking on the phone wasn't the same as being with her. With exams coming up, she was nervous about doing well. School had offered to let her take them later, but she declined, not wanting to have to explain to anyone why she wasn't taking them during the regular exam period. She still struggled with being shy and not wanting to have attention drawn to herself. She also didn't want pity or people she didn't really know asking her questions. She would handle what she was facing, but in her own way and on her own time.

Mike and Caitlin's visit on Wednesday evening had helped cheer Hannah and reassure Caitlin. I had been glad they were there after Hannah started to do a little better. I had found it hard to see her so ill, and I was used to seeing critically ill patients. My experience gave me the advantage of being able to recognize the difference between recovery secondary to surgery and a possible worsening of her condition from the cancer. Even though she still hadn't been out of bed except to sit for a minute or two in a chair while I changed the sheets, she had started to eat a little and looked less pale and drawn.

We also received the results of the HLA testing, which would affect

Caitlin a lot. To our surprise, she was a 5 out of 6 match and could be Hannah's bone marrow donor if and when we reached that point. As Dr. Schwenn explained, this was an excellent match, and she was surprised that with only one sibling this had happened. My children were more alike than even I had known. It gave me some hope, but it also added to my stress. I knew it would help Caitlin feel good because she could help Hannah, but I didn't want her to feel she *had* to do it. Still, if she didn't want to, how would one deal with that? We could only cross one bridge at a time. First the chemotherapy had to put Hannah in remission.

This had been the longest seven days of my life, ones I hoped never to have to repeat. With Hannah doing better, the hectic pace of her care had slowed; she was even a bit restless. So I was pleased when Hannah's piano teacher called to ask if she could come to see us in the hospital. We gladly said yes, and Hannah's spirits rose in anticipation of a visitor. Andrea was not only a friend, but also a mentor to Hannah. She loved seeing Hannah progress in classical piano. In the past, she had worked as an ICU nurse for many years, so we had much in common. I was enjoying seeing her, but had a favor to ask: I needed a break and wanted a chance to take a walk. She was delighted to stay with Hannah while I went out.

Once more, I walked through the streets of the Western Promenade. The exercise felt good. It was debilitating being confined in a hospital room. The only time I stretched my legs was when I went downstairs to the cafeteria. To increase the effect, I walked down seven flights of stairs and then back up. Once outside, I thought I would really enjoy being away for a bit, but my enjoyment was short-lived. I couldn't keep my mind from working overtime imagining things going wrong while I was away. I turned back toward the hospital after only about ten minutes. I knew I couldn't prevent every possible complication, but if I wasn't there, my fears said anything could happen.

Hannah was sleeping when I returned and I breathed a sigh of relief that my fears were unfounded. I relaxed as I joined Andrea on the couch and settled down to chat.

Suddenly, Hannah turned over in bed, sat up and yelled, "Mom, I'm bleeding!"

I grabbed tissues, ran to her bed, and pressed the nurse call button. Blood was all over her pillow and her hand, and her left nostril was dripping blood. I applied pressure under her nose to slow the bleeding.

The combination of the drying effect of the oxygen and the nasal cannula prong putting pressure on the inside of Hannah's nose had caused the bleed. With pressure and cold compresses, the bleeding eventually stopped, but my heart rate didn't slow much as I thought about how a fairly simple problem such as a nosebleed could become a major medical crisis. What had been only a theoretical concern became a reality. Even though Hannah had been receiving transfusions of platelets, her platelet count was still low and she was very susceptible to bleeding.

Gail, Hannah's nurse for the day, reassured us they were watching her closely for this type of complication and would continue to give her platelet transfusions to prevent severe bleeding problems. She placed a container of sterile water between the oxygen-flow gauge and the tubing to her nose to moisturize the oxygen. This would decrease the drying effect and hopefully she wouldn't continue to have nosebleeds. The possibility of uncontrolled bleeding from a low platelet count was a part of cancer treatment that I knew about but had not yet consciously applied to Hannah. Now, it would become another automatic part of daily assessment for me.

Andrea helped Hannah clean up while I changed her bed. Hannah had been frightened by waking up bleeding, and I was glad to have Andrea's calm support. After she left, my thoughts turned to the fear I had experienced when I was out walking. I convinced myself I was being overly cautious, but now it would be hard to let my guard down again any time soon.

After lunch, Gail came in to tell us Hannah would be moved into the smaller of the two positive-pressure rooms on the unit. These rooms worked by having a powerful airflow out of the room so that germs weren't able to easily come in. Even though her blood counts and ability to fight infection were not yet severely diminished, they wanted her there.

This smaller room had windows facing out over the Portland Seadogs baseball stadium and part of Deering Oaks Park. Her new room was on the other side of the teen room, but still across from the nurse's station. While it was great to be so close to the nurse's station while she was so very ill, as Hannah began to improve, it was less exciting to hear the telephones ringing and the staff conversations. Hannah seemed oblivious to it all, but I found it harder to cope with. I hoped when I came back on Sunday night I would make a better adjustment to living in her room.

Because she was doing so well with her recovery from surgery, and despite our scare with the nosebleed, it seemed positively restful to *only* worry about things like preventing complications from the chemotherapy. Of course these new enemies could be deadly as well. Stomatitis (sores or infection of her mouth or digestive tract), ulcerations of her eyes, bowel rupture or bladder problems, bleeding of any kind, and a central-line infection were all very real possibilities. These were not trivial, and preventing them would be as crucial to her survival as having the chemotherapy.

For Hannah, the eye drops, mouthwashes, oxygen saturation monitor on her finger, and the nasal cannula in her nose were all annoying, but she tolerated them. I went over with her the importance of preventive care as a part of getting well. She was very compliant and did very little complaining, but all of the small annoyances still affected her. We tried to maintain a routine that had times when none of the unpleasant parts of her care were being done.

It was a hard thing to make an ill child do something unpleasant or difficult, but because I knew what could happen if it wasn't done, it became like many other difficult parent tasks. We did what we had to do. One very big concern was that she still had her braces which put her at very high risk of mouth sores and infection. If this happened, it could greatly complicate the treatment process, especially if she couldn't eat. While an infection in her mouth wouldn't be immediately life-threatening, it would make her miserable and wasn't worth the risk. We strictly adhered to the schedule for mouthwashes and using the Water Pik even though she hated doing them.

Before I left, I wanted to have everything set up and in place so Mike wouldn't have to worry about her care; he could just enjoy the time he would have with her. Once we had completed the move into her new room, I gathered all I needed to take home and packed my bag. Even though it was late in the evening, I was not comfortable leaving until Mike arrived. Not only did I want to see him and explain what he needed to be aware of in her care, but I also worried something might happen if I left her alone again. I trusted the nurses who were working that night, but if something were to happen after I left and before Mike arrived, I would always blame myself.

Mike was exhausted from work and his long drive, but very happy to see Hannah doing better. Even though he had been there on Wednesday, it seemed as if I hadn't seen him for a long time. I just wanted to be with him. Coping with our feelings by phone was very hard, and at this point, we had no idea when we could be together again for any length of time.

So many emotional ups and downs, so many physical changes; it was almost impossible to believe how radically our lives had changed in so short a time. One week ago we were preparing to go to the Memorial Day soccer tournament with no thoughts other than wondering if Hannah's soccer team would play well and have a good record in the tournament.

Now my only worry was that my daughter could still die, and I couldn't imagine ever caring about a soccer tournament again. My world had narrowed to a hospital room, my family, and Hannah's survival.

The closer to home I got, the more excited I became. I couldn't wait to see Caitlin and hear about her week, plus the thought of sleeping in my own bed without the noise and hospital smells was thrilling. Getting up in the night to go to the bathroom would be a private experience. Wow! It was amazing what simple things made me happy now.

Caitlin and I snuggled up on the couch, the dog resting on my feet on the floor. He was feeling the strain just like the rest of us. Because Caitlin hadn't told any of her friends at school about what was happening, she had carried a heavy burden alone all week. As always, the dance of motherhood required listening more than telling. As she unburdened herself, I realized she had assumed many of the tasks of running the house while I was away. She didn't complain about being left on her own or the extra responsibility. We had not discussed her needing to do it, but she had undertaken this role without question. I was also poignantly aware of her new role as Hannah's potential donor. It made her feel very good that she could do something so important to help Hannah.

I looked down at her as she leaned on my shoulder and saw her in a new way. She had taken one of those giant "growing-up leaps" kids do when you're not looking.

"Caitlin, I know how hard this week has been for you. I'm so proud of how you've handled all of this. It really helped Hannah when you came on Wednesday. She perked right up."

"She didn't look as bad as I was afraid she would," she said.

"Hannah really looks up to you, and if you are positive about what's happening, it will help her."

"Mom, Hannah is going to beat this. She can't die!"

"Oh, sweetie, I hope you're right. I really want to believe she won't."

I hugged her tightly as we sat in silence. I sensed something else was bothering her, but didn't want to push too hard. As we walked upstairs arm in arm, she stopped outside my room, reluctant to let go.

"Is something else bothering you?" I asked.

"We had a dress-down day at school. It was a fundraiser for cancer research. You know the boy in my class whose mother died of cancer? Well, the Upper School was honoring her with this donation in her name."

"Were you really upset because it was cancer?"

"Partly. I only had a dollar because I didn't know about it ahead of time, but they also asked us to have a moment of silence to think about anyone we knew who had cancer."

"Oh, sweetie, that must have been so hard for you."

"Mom, I cried and I was so embarrassed. I couldn't tell anyone why I was crying. I just don't want people feeling sorry for me. People I don't even know would be saying things to me. It's nobody else's business. I can't talk about it because I might cry."

"Oh, Caitlin. You don't need to be embarrassed about how you're feeling. I'm certain there were lots of people who cried. I would have been bawling my eyes out. Isn't there even one friend you can talk to who won't bug you about it?"

"I'm just not ready to do that, Mom."

"When you're ready, I think it will be easier for you if you have someone who can just be supportive. Would it make you feel better to take in a bigger donation on Monday? I can give you money for a donation if it would help you feel better. Or we could send a donation to the American Cancer Society in her name."

"I'll think about it."

I walked her to her room and tucked her into bed. I didn't know how to help her other than to listen and love, but it hurt that she was in pain and I wasn't able to be there for her.

Alone again, I dragged myself back to my room, a yoke of exhaustion on my neck and shoulders. Even when I thought I was doing okay, fear crept up and gave me a jolt. I wanted to beg for something less demanding. Not having that as a choice, I returned to putting one foot in front of the other, forcing myself to move forward.

As I brushed my teeth, the person I saw in the mirror looked the same, aside from tear stains and red eyes, but I wasn't the person I had been ten days ago. I had a new identity: cancer parent. My family was asunder and emotionally fragile. We had a monumental struggle ahead of us. If Hannah survived, we would all be very different people. Could I ever be that trusting, optimistic person I had been before this started? Could I keep everything together for everyone? I didn't know if I had the strength.

After a day of endless household chores, physical fatigue brought a second night of deep sleep and I felt rested for the first time in weeks. Although it seemed I had just arrived home, the time with Caitlin had flown by. I wanted to defy physics and be in two places at once, but I had to go back. With fresh laundry, some additional books, all the logistical arrangements for Caitlin's week of final exams completed, I braced for another week.

Chapter 11
NEIGHBORS

Community: "It takes a village to raise a child" (African proverb), and it takes a caring community to help a family survive childhood cancer.

On medical rounds, Dr. Schwenn asked if we knew anyone with A negative blood. They were having trouble getting platelets for Hannah, and because the cancer and chemo destroyed them, she needed transfusions every few days to help with blood-clotting. Without them, bleeding could be as fatal as not treating the cancer. What ensued was one of those things which restored my faith in the community of man.

I called friends in York, Maine, where we used to live, and at Hannah's school, and then sent an e-mail to our good friend Kelly Martin, assistant women's soccer coach at UNH. Having known Hannah through summer soccer camps since Hannah was in kindergarten, Kelly was devastated by the news of her diagnosis and cared deeply about helping with anything she could.

Within an hour, the phone rang and a man said, "Is this Carol Glover?"

"Yes, it is. May I help you?".

"You don't know me, but my niece works at UNH and she just called me to say some little girl needs A negative platelets. She knows I'm A negative, so I'm calling. What do you need me to do?"

I was so surprised I had received a response so quickly; I almost didn't know what to say.

"Thank you. I'm the little girl's mother, her name is Hannah, and we do need platelets. We're at Maine Medical Center in Portland."

"Well, I'm only about a half hour from there; where do I donate?"

I gave him the information I had been given and thanked him profusely for his help and kindness. It was the first of several calls from home, Cape Elizabeth, York, and a few other Maine towns. At one point there were so many people wanting to donate platelets that the blood collection service sent a mobile unit to our town rather than have people from New Hampshire travel to Scarborough, Maine. Interestingly, four teachers at Hannah's school were A negative. They made T-shirts celebrating their donations.

Throughout the rest of the time Hannah was being treated, I had people whom I didn't know stopping me in our local grocery store to ask if we still needed platelets. We never again were at risk of not being able to get them for Hannah, and the local blood drives had a lot of new donors for this rarer type of blood.

It had always been hard for me to ask for help. I was used to being the one giving it, but now, for Hannah's sake, I was willing to beg if need be. Fortunately, we had so much help I didn't always know what to tell people we needed. Food and rides for Caitlin to her activities and visits to the hospital were the highest on my list. Several friends helped with the dog, including veterinary visits and walks. For the most part, anything we needed was available, but it still felt strange to be in such need.

Friends who owned a local shop called the Bagelry set up an e-mail list so I could send one e-mail for mass distribution. Mike had done the same for a family list. Thank goodness for e-mail, the Internet, and cheap prepaid phone cards. They made getting help or giving updates on Hannah much easier.

Since school was still in session, Hannah had very few visitors. I was concerned she might feel abandoned by her friends as she traveled down a path none of them would (hopefully) ever follow. Would she begin to feel alienated from their experiences, and would she lose the commonality of experience which makes surviving the teen years possible? There had been no news of how long she would be in the hospital, and with no end in sight, she could become depressed and discouraged.

That problem was partially alleviated by a visit from Hannah's teacher, John Silverio, and the classroom intern. They brought cards and messages from her classmates which she posted around her room. They told her stories of what was going on in school and how projects in the classroom were going. It boosted her spirits and relieved some of the boredom.

While we were isolated from our home community, we had a new community in the hospital. It included mostly the medical and nursing staff at this point. Their constant care was essential, and we were slowly getting to know them as individuals. Hannah still couldn't sit up for any length of time or walk to the bathroom, but she was improving. She no longer looked like my bubbly, energetic kid, but she was laughing and talking about the weekend. She had color in her face and her breathing was stable. I realized I was slowly changing my norms; compared to her healthy self, she looked terrible, but for this moment she wasn't having trouble breathing and didn't have a fever. Every moment she wasn't in crisis was a moment for joy.

The nurse cares for multiple patients with a variety of needs, and allots time based on how acutely ill each patient is. Because I understood the normal hospital routines and why they were done, I expected I would be more tolerant of what they needed to do, but I became as self-absorbed as any other parent in putting Hannah's needs first.

I was so relieved by how much better Hannah was and about getting the platelets, I was able to fall into the deepest sleep of any night since admission. Unfortunately, our community of nurses had a new member on duty who, when she came in to do Hannah's care, startled me awake by touching my shoulder. I sat bolt upright with my heart pounding as I immediately assumed the worst. Instead, she just wanted to introduce herself and let me know she would be on duty until morning.

I'm certain she was attempting to be courteous and professional, but being awakened to have introductions was not high on my priority list. In fact, my first thought when I realized there was nothing wrong with Hannah was more along the lines of homicide. I later came to appreciate her excellent nursing competence, but the ability to function quietly was not one of her best attributes. I never told her how lucky she was to have survived that night.

I knew from research studies that the effects of sleep disruption can be very detrimental to healing and recovery. Most nursing departments now try to bundle night nursing care so there are fewer sleep interruptions. I spoke with the night nurses about the possibility of doing that, as long as Hannah wasn't critical, and they were very receptive.

Meeting new people continued the next day on rounds. Our nurse, Kristen, told us we would be meeting Dr. Craig Hurwitz, the head of the MCCP oncology team. She told us he was back from his conference and vacation and that Hannah would love him. Hannah looked a little skeptical, but said, "Okay," in her "I'll wait and see voice."

A few minutes later Dr. Hurwitz entered the room and in a Texas drawl tinged with many years in Maine, he said, "My, oh, my. You're even more beautiful than they told me you were. I'm Craig Hurwitz."

As he shook her hand and smiled, she giggled and melted into answering smiles.

"Hi. I'm Hannah."

I don't know if it was love at first sight, but there was definitely a mutual admiration society being formed. In a very short visit during rounds, he managed to elicit a lot of information from her, including that she played classical piano. After admitting he was learning to play the fiddle, he told her he would make certain she got a keyboard to continue her piano practicing while she was in the hospital. Her spirits rose and I think for the first time she anticipated something more than feeling sick and being confined in this small isolation room. I don't remember the rest of that conversation; I was too busy being grateful that Hannah so clearly trusted and enjoyed this team of physicians into whose hands we had entrusted her life.

As the week progressed, there was a rhythm to the day and night. My sleep came at night between the vital signs checks, but was disrupted all too frequently by IV pump alarms or phones ringing at the nurse's station outside our room. Sleep during the day came in the form of short naps if Hannah was resting or asleep after medication for a transfusion or treatment. In these naps and my nighttime sleep, I slept so deeply from exhaustion, I awoke disoriented. There was still always that one brief moment between sleep and waking when I didn't remember what had happened. As awareness crashed back in with a heart-thumping jolt, I immediately checked to see if Hannah was okay. When she was, I felt relieved, and after taking several deep breaths and willing my heart rate to return to normal, I tried to return to sleep, sometimes with success, but more often without.

Each day, Hannah was becoming stronger, and was able to sit in a chair or walk to and from the bathroom. She was feeling so much better she was starting to be bored.

It was a welcome surprise at rounds on Wednesday when Bethany, the MCCP Nurse Practitioner said, "Are you ready to head home for a few days to get Hannah's braces off and have some time away from here? We've decided it would be easier to have her own orthodontist do the work than to have an orthodontist from here come in to do it."

I was excited by the prospect, but also confused and a little panicked at the notion I would be allowed to take such a sick child home.

"Uh, are we allowed to take her out of the positive-pressure room, and what do we need to do to take her home? Are her counts okay? Will she be at high risk at home?"

"Her counts are still okay, and as long as she isn't exposed to too many people, she should be fine. She will be okay with her own home environment, but it might be a good idea to get extra stuffed animals and books out of her room. You will need a place to set up a sterile field for her dressing changes and for flushing her central line ports," Bethany said.

"Uh, we can do that."

I couldn't quite take in that we would be going home so soon. I was excited, but at the same time, I was worried. Was it safe? What would we do about blood work? Where would we get dressing supplies? Was her room safe for her to be in since her blood counts were still decreasing daily? Were there any special concerns for which we should be prepared? When would we need to return?

I realized that Bethany had done this many times before. She had answers for most of my questions without my even asking.

"We'll have all of the referrals and supplies before you leave. We'll arrange the referral for Critical Care Systems in your area to draw blood and check on her central line while she is at home, and we want her to have her braces removed as soon as possible. We'll schedule the appointment for Monday. You'll need to be checked off by the nurses here to change her central line dressings and flush her lines with heparinized saline. That shouldn't be a problem for you, right?" she said.

"I hope not," I said.

"You should be ready to go by Friday, if she doesn't develop a fever or have any other problems."

"When will Critical Care Systems come?" I asked.

"The day you get home or the next day, depending on when you leave here. We will set it all up before you leave. You do understand that this will all depend on Hannah staying fever-free for the next day or so?"

"Yes, I do, and thank you so much."

She was very matter-of-fact about what was, for me, a major change. What might seem to the medical staff the next logical step came as a surprise to us. Perhaps they thought I would know this, but I hadn't thought beyond what we did each hour of the day. Taking Hannah home seemed a very big responsibility. I wanted to be away from the hospital, but at the same time, I knew that her counts would be going down and that she would be at risk for infection and other possible complications. Would I recognize what was happening in time? Were there things unique to childhood cancer I didn't know about and might have problems with?

As soon as Dr. Hamilton, another of the MCCP oncologists, finished examining Hannah and our part of rounds was over, Hannah and I talked about the exciting news. Even though she was happy about the prospect, I sensed she was also a little nervous. Since admission, there had always been nurses and doctors available twenty-four hours a day. Even though she trusted I would be there, she hadn't been away from medical care since her diagnosis.

"Are you worried about being home without the medical people around?"

"Well, maybe a little bit," she answered.

"We'll have everything we need for your central lines, dressings, and heparin flushes, and they'll send a visiting nurse from Critical Care Systems to check on everything."

"Oh, I'm not worried about that. I don't know if I can get used to sleeping at home without being woken up every few hours," she said and gave a big laugh.

"Very funny! Here I am worrying about getting your room ready and all of that and you're a comedian."

She giggled again and gave me an "Oh, Mom" look.

"It will work out, Mom, don't worry."

Who was the parent and who was the child? I thought.

Mike reacted as I had when I called to tell him. Would she be all right at home, and was she ready to leave the hospital? I shared with him all that Bethany and Dr. Hamilton had explained to me. He was reassured and then grateful he wouldn't have to drive all the way to Portland on Friday, but we both knew this could all change in an instant if she had a fever.

When I called Caitlin, I let Hannah tell her. From what I could hear as they chattered excitedly, this was welcome news. I asked Caitlin if she could clean Hannah's room if I got someone else to be there to help her. She was eager to do whatever it took to get ready for Hannah to be home.

I contacted the help list, and my friend Patty, a fellow Nurse Practitioner, called to say she would be happy come over to work with Caitlin. The next day, they took everything out of Hannah's room, packed up books, stuffed animals, and extraneous items, and washed down everything with disinfectant cleaner. It was a big job and I was very grateful for the help.

Once her room was ready, we only had to have the good luck of not developing a fever, but I had one other concern: summer had started in earnest and we didn't own an air conditioner. I was worried that Hannah might develop fever problems just from being overheated at home. In the hospital, she insisted on having the thermostat in her room set at 58 or 60 degrees. The nurses frequently tried to turn it up, but she really felt better with the room cold. I dealt with it by dressing warmly and sleeping with extra blankets.

I wanted to purchase an air conditioner, but since it had been so hot, most places had already sold out. To my surprise and gratitude, I received an e-mail saying that, since the word was out that Hannah might be able to come home, a family in the community wanted to lend us a window air conditioner for as long as we needed it. I was amazed at their generosity and questioned whether they wouldn't be miserable without it. They assured me they had several and their children could share a cooled room if they needed to. My belief that we had chosen the best possible place to live if you had to go through this was being confirmed.

The next time Disey came in to change Hannah's central line dressing, I asked if it would be a good time for me to be observed flushing her central line and changing the dressing. She was ready to let me proceed immediately. I felt a little nervous; not only had it been a while since I had changed a central line dressing, but this was my child. Hannah and I both put on masks and I laid out a sterile field for the dressing change. I took a deep breath and mentally distanced myself from whose body this dressing and central line was on. It came off without a hitch and one obstacle to heading home was removed.

Luck was with us; Hannah didn't develop a fever. We were packed and ready to leave by the time all of the paperwork and referrals were done. It felt as if she had been hospitalized for a lifetime. In reality she had. We were no longer the individuals or family we were when we walked through the doors of Admitting. Our lives were completely altered, and now we only saw the world from the perspective of a cancer family. We had entered a new world, a new way of life. It felt as if we belonged to an exclusive club with secret code signals. If you weren't a member, you would never understand them, but if you were, you immediately recognized a fellow traveler. Even though we would shortly be returning for the second part of the first round of chemotherapy, I was overjoyed that for the next several days we would all be together in one place.

Chapter 12
BALD AND BEYOND

*Alopecia medicamentosa: diffuse hair loss, most notably of the scalp,
but may also include eyebrows, eyelashes, and body hair, caused by
administration of various drugs, especially chemotherapy agents.*

We were home! Even though I got up every few hours to touch Hannah to check for a fever, examine the central line clamps to see that they were still closed, and listen to her steady breathing, I felt as if I were on vacation. We were together in one place and Hannah was still alive! I was sleeping in my own bed and I could, for a few minutes at a time, not think about what we had endured in the past two weeks or what we were still facing in the future.

When we left the hospital on Friday, six days at home seemed an eternity. Hannah was very nearly her old self, happy to be away from constant intrusions into her privacy. The first couple of nights, we discovered that both Hannah and I were awakening at the times vital signs were normally checked. Fortunately, going back to sleep wasn't a problem. It still seemed strange that only a couple of weeks ago she was so ill she couldn't sit up, but was now okay to be at home without being continuously monitored. The Critical Care nurse had approved our sterile technique for flushing the central line ports and changing the central line dressing. We kept a strict schedule for checking her temperature and the care of her central line.

The orthodontist had removed her braces on Monday, and their staff had provided Hannah such a huge basket of goodies we had to go out the back door so that other patients wouldn't be jealous. We had to spend all of Tuesday on our first trip to MCCP in Scarborough to see Dr. Schwenn in the clinic. Hannah's platelet count was very low, so they gave her a transfusion. While we were there, we met the clinic staff and learned the protocol for receiving care in the clinic versus the hospital.

Now, with only one more day at home, we were preparing for our return to the hospital. However, there was one more treat in store.

Hannah's teacher brought a group of students from her class bearing gifts and messages from everyone. As I sat in the background watching her laughing and giggling with friends, I could feel tears threatening to leak out. I was heartbroken that she would never again belong to this innocent world of preadolescence. Things I had worried most about for her, like social pressures and academic challenges, now seemed simple.

The students were initially shy and tentative, but once they realized she was still Hannah, they all talked excitedly about what was happening at school. She was happy and I wanted to be able to just enjoy it, but instead I worried one of them might be getting sick with something that Hannah could catch. I was sad but relieved when they left. I was also jealous. Their world seemed so simple, so unthreatening, while Hannah's was filled with danger and even possible death. I still had acceptance issues.

It was confining and more than a little depressing to move back into the small positive-pressure room. We brought decorations and more stuffed animals, but it wasn't home. Our admission nurse, Gail, congratulated us on making it through all six days, since a fever often brought a patient back sooner. Perhaps naively, I hadn't worried about that. Except that she was tired, Hannah was more normal than she had been in the six weeks prior to her diagnosis and admission. It was tempting to say, "Let's quit now while she is feeling so much better; not take the chance of complications making things worse," but I knew better.

As soon as she was finished with the admission, preparation for chemotherapy began. By late afternoon, after the IV antinausea medication, eye drops, and medicated mouthwashes were administered, she had a dose of ARA-C and the consolidation phase of the first round of chemotherapy was underway. She lay curled up in a ball under her blue, fuzzy kitty blanket, Lovey Bear under her head, surrounded by her other stuffed animals, all of the liveliness of the last few days gone.

There wasn't much to do, so I did what made me feel better. I organized all our things in drawers and closets and made space for the new addition to our room, an extra over-bed tray table on which sat an electric keyboard. Dr. Hurwitz had followed through. Now Hannah could play piano when she felt well enough. Even though she didn't do it often, it was a reminder that she could.

Weight loss during chemotherapy can be a major complication. At home, Hannah had eaten very well because she liked what I cooked, but here she didn't like a lot of the food. She understood that if she couldn't keep her weight up, she would have to receive TPN (total parenteral nutrition, an intravenous solution that provides full nutrients) via her central line. This would mean staying in the hospital even when her blood counts would otherwise allow her to return home.

I talked with her about the need to make eating, just like drinking a lot of water, a part of treatment as if it were a medication or a procedure. Even if she didn't have much of an appetite, she understood how important it was. Fortunately, she craved certain high-calorie foods like McDonald's bacon, egg, and cheese biscuits. I would normally consider this junk food, but their high calorie count made them a good choice for regaining some weight. To provide her with these sandwiches, I combined a four-mile early morning walk with a trip to the McDonald's restaurant we could see from our window. When I returned around 6:30 or 7:00, she was usually awake and ready to eat. This would have been expensive except instead of eating in the cafeteria, I ate the boiled egg, fruit, and bagel that she ordered for breakfast. The nutritionist made a clinical visit to us because she thought Hannah was eating low-calorie meals. We had gotten caught in our deception.

Familiarity with the staff and hospital routines, and being less critically ill made Hannah more comfortable with being an inpatient, but now she was bored whenever she wasn't feeling ill. I realized that unless we worked at it, her room could become our whole world. My morning walk got me out of the room, but she could only escape through television or books. It was hard to keep a supply of books and videos. The Child Life staff, trained in play therapy, provided many activities in the playroom and made every effort to help with this problem, but it was still frustrating.

Besides walking, and an occasional trip downstairs to the main cafeteria or the chapel, I stayed in her room or on the unit. Because it was a closed world, it was easy to narrow our interactions down to those people who were also living there. The only new acquaintances I made were other families whose children were seriously ill.

One of the nurses introduced me to the mother of the child next door in the other positive-pressure room. Before she introduced us, the nurse explained that the child had been diagnosed with AML a year previous, was Hannah's age, and had been in remission after the initial five rounds of chemotherapy. Unfortunately, almost exactly a year after the initial diagnosis, he relapsed and treatment had to be resumed to regain remission. The next step would be a bone marrow transplant, if they could find a donor. Without a transplant his chance of survival was dismal. She thought it might help his mother to talk with someone who would understand her feelings.

In my professional life, I was a giver, finding it easy to interact with and reach out to those I provided care for. Now, I could barely cope with our situation, and felt superstitious about not wanting to know what other children and families had experienced. Logic to the contrary, not knowing felt as if it would somehow protect Hannah from any of the complications they faced in their battles with cancer.

The two positive-pressure rooms shared an anteroom with a sink and cabinets where gowns and supplies were kept. I had seen this mother, but we had only nodded in passing. It felt as if we were in nonintersecting isolation bubbles of misery.

After the introduction, we talked standing outside our respective rooms. Her child had an infection, and until it was treated, they couldn't go to Dana Farber for a transplant. Exhaustion rode her shoulders and her shadow-ringed eyes had a cornered, hunted look in them. As she talked about their treatment experiences, her voice betrayed a hopelessness born of months of fighting this battle and not winning.

We exchanged offerings of sympathy, but no words were adequate. She opened the door to their room and I caught a momentary glimpse inside. My stomach turned at the sight of this young boy curled up on the bed, ashen-faced, with dark circles surrounding large eyes full of pain. I didn't need my experience to understand how ill this child was. A wave of nausea and lightheadedness swept through me. Would Hannah reach this state? His cancer was advanced before treatment began, with a high tumor load and generalized bruising, but this rationalization didn't make me feel any less frightened.

I had been hopeful because Hannah seemed to be tolerating this phase of chemotherapy easily. Now I realized she had probably just been lucky to have been home for those few days and responding to treatment. I couldn't imagine this family's despair at a relapse now, after completing chemo and being in remission for nearly a year.

For weeks afterwards, when I couldn't sleep, I obsessed over my conversation with the mother and the images of her son, aware of what could happen in cancer treatment. I wished I hadn't talked with her about their experiences. I wanted to believe Hannah would do well. Neither cancer nor the complications were catching, but I understood for the first time how easily people became superstitiously afraid of someone with a life-threatening illness.

A couple of days later, I met another family with a five-year-old daughter with AML. They were in the hospital now because of an infection. We exchanged stories and felt a connection because they were both health care professionals. They had been at home preparing to return for another round of chemo when she developed a fever requiring emergency admission. I had yet to fully understand firsthand the fear of infections and complications which everyone in the cancer world has, but I was learning.

When I didn't see them on the unit the next morning, I thought perhaps she had been discharged. As I was returning from my shower, I was surprised to see the parents in the corridor. They looked as if they hadn't slept in weeks. Concerned, I asked them what was happening. The answer was not good. Their daughter was in the Pediatric Intensive Care Unit (PICU) in a medically induced coma to control pain from the fluid building up around her brain, a complication of the infection. A shunt would be needed to drain the fluid, and they wouldn't know until after the infection was controlled and the coma was reversed, if there would be permanent brain damage. How could they be standing there so calmly talking with me? Why weren't they hysterical? I wanted to run away and not hear more, but I stayed and listened knowing they probably needed to tell someone who might understand.

The number of things that could go wrong from a combination of treatment complications and an imunno-compromised state (low white blood cell counts which keep the immune system from being able to fight infection) seemed infinite. How could anyone have hope and keep going with this feeling of a guillotine swinging over your head all the time? These parents seemed so courageous. I wondered if I could be that strong if Hannah developed complications. As they hurried back to the PICU, I became very anxious about Hannah and walked quickly back to her room to reassure myself that she was still okay. It was certainly easier to work long hours as a nurse caring for people you didn't know than to do this.

Since we had returned to the hospital on a Thursday, I would be able to go home while Mike was with Hannah for the weekend. The chemotherapy would continue until Tuesday. Having seen the effects of secondary complications from infections, I was determined to be even more vigilant in enforcing preventive measures. I talked with Hannah about how important it was to use her mouth rinse at the scheduled times, not resist having the eye drops instilled in her eyes, and to stay well hydrated and continue to eat well.

I did one additional thing before I left. I had noticed some hair on Hannah's pillow and realized it would probably begin to fall out more rapidly as she finished this part of chemo. Even though Disey had talked with us about it, Hannah wasn't showing much concern, so I didn't make a fuss about it. I did, however, wash and braid her hair. Compared with all of the possible pitfalls and complications, I suddenly didn't feel hair loss would be the worst thing that could happen.

After a refreshing weekend at home with Caitlin, I was eager to see Hannah, but I stopped short when I opened her door and looked into her room. Mike and Hannah had clearly had a very relaxing weekend. My concerns about neatness and a strict hospital routine had not ranked high on their list of priorities. Her braid had come undone, her hair hadn't been washed, and now there was a huge bird's nest of tangled, wadded hair on the back of her head. I bit my lip to keep from crying.

After I hugged Hannah and then Mike, I asked, "Why didn't you keep Hannah's hair combed and braided?"

He turned away, but not before I saw his tears.

"It's starting to come out in handfuls. I wanted to leave it there as long as possible."

I swallowed my own tears, unable to say anything else. He was having a very hard time coping with this symbol of Hannah's cancer, but I felt resentful that this had fallen to me to take care of. I didn't want to upset Hannah, so I let it go.

After Mike left, I talked with Hannah about getting the tangles out of her hair. She hadn't wanted a haircut before, but now she agreed she couldn't keep it combed. It was all over her pillow and she didn't like that. With a pair of bandage scissors, I cut out the tangled mess and gave her a short haircut that framed her face. It looked very cute and was easier to care for.

I don't know how she really felt about losing her prized long blond hair, but she was pleased with her haircut and handled it like so many other things; if it couldn't be changed, she would just live with it. I marveled at her ability to cope without complaint. Needing to shed my tears in private, I gathered the dirty clothes and headed to the laundry area.

I thought about other cancer patients I had known who involved their families and communities in head-shaving parties where solidarity in baldness was established. Hannah didn't want to shave her head before her hair fell out, and we were not in a "celebrating hair loss" mood, so we let it happen *to* us. For me, it was the symbol of another line crossed as we slipped further into the world of cancer treatment.

Even though Hannah said she wasn't upset about losing her hair, she did want a wig. The next day, Liz, our social worker, helped us set up a meeting with the "wig lady." Before all of Hannah's hair fell out, the color and texture needed to be matched to samples of hair for wigs. Disey tried to convince Hannah that she probably wouldn't need a wig, but Hannah really wanted one to wear when she wanted to be out and about at home. Until she had a wig, the stylish and colorful summer hats that friends and family had given her were enough.

Hannah was excited about the wig fitting. The woman who came was the picture of a well-groomed, genteel middle-aged lady. Her hair was a perfect dome without a strand out of place. I looked twice and then hoped it wasn't a wig. Her work could not have been easy. Unfortunately, she was mushily sentimental about "this poor lamb with cancer." As she discussed wig styles and hair color, she measured Hannah's head and tried to pat and cluck over her terrible fate. Hannah shied away. I quickly ran interference by asking questions about insurance coverage so that Hannah could choose a style that she liked unfettered by sympathy. If it had not been such a sensitive subject, I could have laughed, but the laughter caught in my throat and threatened to dissolve into tears. I didn't want this to be traumatic for Hannah; losing her hair was bad enough. I also didn't want to upset this well-meaning lady.

I stood beside Hannah while she narrowed down her selection and focused on how she could style her wig while it was off her head. Hannah burst out laughing as I described how hard I had always found it to do anything with my hair and wished I could take it off. By using my body to maintain a comfortable personal space for Hannah, she came to a decision. I carefully herded the woman out of the room and finished the discussion of pickup and business details in the hall.

The wig saga continued on an extremely hot day when we were due to pick it up from the shop. Friends who had moved to upstate New York were back for a visit and had brought Caitlin with them to the hospital. Katie was a year older than Hannah and Julia was Caitlin's age and they all got along well. It was the first time we had seen them since they'd moved. Hannah's blood counts were still high enough for her to be out on a pass, so we decided to have a picnic on the Eastern Promenade after picking up the wig. At the shop all four girls were in a great mood as they admired all of the wigs, scarves, and prosthetics in the store. The other girls all wanted to try on and style Hannah's wig, which made it special for her. As Disey had predicted, Hannah never really wore her wig that much, but she had the option.

By the time most of her hair was gone and only a few wispy strands remained, I had grown to love her bald head. It was soft and I felt nothing but tenderness each time I saw it. She tolerated my need to kiss and touch her head occasionally, but didn't want me making a fuss. She hadn't been willing to talk much about it, but wasn't depressed. I think she coped with this like many other things. It was a part of what was going to happen and being upset wouldn't make it go away.

A few days after our wig adventure, her counts dropped rapidly and we were no longer able to leave on pass. The isolation room now represented the extent of Hannah's world. The only clue I had that she wasn't feeling good about it was that she refused to leave her room even though, as long as she wore a mask, she could. The mask made her feel self-conscious. She refused to go to the playroom or the teen room even though she had been enjoying doing so. Finally, someone else intervened to help her.

For her room to be cleaned and mopped, they opened the big hallway door, which gave Hannah a view of the nurse's station. She sat cross-legged on her bed, mask in place. A boy about her age peeked around the door frame. He too was wearing a mask.

"Come play video games with me in the teen room. I don't have anybody to play with!"

Hannah hesitated.

"Why don't you go? He has to wear a mask as well. Take a chance. It might be fun."

Reluctantly she pulled her robe on, found her slippers, and followed him next door to the teen room. He wanted to play a video car-chase game, and soon they were racing. I stood outside the door and felt the now all-too-familiar lump form in my throat. With their IV pumps and poles behind them, their bald heads side by side, and their masks making them look like they were participating in some strange costume drama, they dueled it out; just two kids having fun.

Afterwards, whenever she was bored and not feeling bad, she left the room to walk around or play in the playroom. I was grateful to this young boy who helped Hannah feel okay about leaving her room and interacting with other people. It broke the ice for her and they became friends so that whenever they were both in the hospital and were able to, they played together.

Chapter 13
ARRAY

Gamut: the entire range of something;
from crisis to boredom and back again.

Our days now seemed to resemble the description by an airline pilot about his job. Flying is mostly a pretty boring and easy job unless you are taking off or landing, a warning light goes on, or alarms sound; then it is pure terror. So far during this admission, our only unexpected pure terror moment was at the end of a transfusion. Hannah's friend Keely was visiting and they were having lots of laughs talking about friends from school. I was enjoying having Keely's mom, Skye, as a visitor as well, and wasn't paying close attention to Hannah, but I glanced up as their laughter died down. Hannah was rubbing her neck, fidgeting, and scratching her back. I jumped off the couch when I saw a bright red splotch on her neck. I pulled up her shirt and gasped as I watched half-dollar-sized hives erupt across her back and onto her chest and arms.

Hannah began to cry and yelled, "Mom, it itches!"

"Don't scratch!" I yelled as I ran to the nurse's station.

Gail, her nurse, took one quick look at Hannah, shut off the blood transfusion, started the saline IV, and ran back to the medicine room. Hannah was crying harder, a frightened look in her eyes.

"My throat itches!"

"Try to take deep, slow breaths, sweetie."

I checked her mouth and could see a couple of red areas.

Gail came back with IV Benadryl and started it on rapid infusion.

As the medication took effect, Hannah's breathing slowed and the hives began to disappear. She lay down on her bed as the medicine made her drowsy. I stood beside her holding her hand as she fell asleep, willing my heart to stop pounding. Our fun day and visit were over.

She had received almost 100% of the unit of blood, and in the last few drops must have encountered a protein that triggered the allergic response which could have become a full-blown anaphylactic reaction.

There was no way to anticipate such life-threatening possibilities. Even though she didn't receive transfusions anywhere but in the hospital or the clinic, constant vigilance was required. It was another reminder of how tenuous our hold was on things being under control. Without a quick response, she could have gone into shock and died.

Gail checked on her again and said, "She'll be okay, but from now on she'll need to be pre-medicated with Benadryl and Tylenol before every transfusion."

"That was a huge reaction!" I said.

"Yeah, it's pretty scary when it happens like that, but we caught it in time. Don't worry; we'll be watching her closely," she said.

In the future, Hannah would be asleep during these procedures. It was a trade-off I was very willing to make as I thought about what a close call this had been. Disaster seemed to always be only one step away; the abyss yawned and one tiny misstep could send us pitching over the edge. As if to drive home the point, the next day we faced a different problem.

Even though central line dressing changes had become "routine" (as if something so critical could ever be routine), Hannah complained her skin around the line hurt when the dressing was removed. The clear dressing material allowed the site to be seen and evaluated every day without having to break sterility, but protocol required the area to be cleaned and new sterile dressing applied every three days. Now she had a reddened, irritated area under the dressing. Since the development of skin sores could be a major complication, this needed to be addressed immediately.

There was a new dressing material that had recently been made available, but it was much more expensive and its use needed prior insurance approval. I wondered if other families, who weren't involved in health care, would even be aware of the process of getting something new approved through insurance. I was weighing the actual cost of the dressing material against the potential cost of skin sores and the complications that could go with them. For me there was no comparison. If we had to pay for it out of pocket, it would be worth the cost. Again we were fortunate: the new material worked once we had the authorization.

We seemed to be in a cycle of good things, bad things. Our nurse, Kristen, came to tell us that the patient in the larger positive-pressure room was leaving for Boston for his bone marrow transplant. We could move into that room with more space, but it meant that going home was not even on the horizon. Hannah's blood counts had almost reached their lowest level of less than 100 white blood cells per millimeter of blood. The chemotherapy had done what it was supposed to do---wipe out her bone marrow---but now she was extremely vulnerable to infection.

Because she could die from an infection as easily as from the cancer, I became rather overbearing about hand-washing to help protect her. I knew it was one of the best defenses against spreading the bacteria and viruses that make us ill. For me, hand-washing was pretty automatic, but I had been around medical personnel long enough to know they might preach this, but didn't always practice it. I carefully watched everyone who came into the room or visited to remind them to use hand sanitizer or, better yet, wash their hands. I was willing to offend to protect Hannah. We had been lucky thus far, so I wasn't taking any unnecessary chances.

After the excitement of moving, Hannah was bored again, so I was thankful when a large package arrived from her teacher. He was trying to keep her a part of what was happening at school. She wouldn't be returning to her classroom and her classmates missed her. Her teacher and several students had started a project in Hannah's honor. At the end-of-school revels, the final Bagel Challenge had been run. The kids had made a picture of a sneaker on five-by-eight sheets of paper then colored or decorated them. Under each sneaker was the slogan, "S miles for Hannah". If the number of sneaker sheets in the boxes we received were any indicator, all 800 students in the school must have participated.

The box also contained a video of the school halls being decorated with the sneaker posters. Some of the students who ran in the Challenge had organized fundraising activities so they could donate to children's cancer research. On the day of the race, a professional videographer had filmed interviews with students who were preparing to run. Many of these students didn't know Hannah personally, but spoke during the interviews about running the race for a 5th grader who had cancer. I realized as I watched the video that Hannah had influenced people she didn't even know. I didn't know how many of these students had ever thought about the idea of working for a cause greater than themselves, but in this situation hundreds of them were doing just that.

Hannah's classmates missed the humorous, kind soul who had been a leader in their class. A second video had messages from all of her classmates and clips from the end-of-the-year dance and celebration she had missed. Students spoke about how she had helped them, was a good friend, or had contributed to the success of various projects they had done during the year. They let her know she was a very special person whom they missed.

Because we hadn't known what was in the package, we weren't prepared for a ten-hankie afternoon. Hannah watched her friends and listened to their messages, read through the sneaker cards, with their get-well notes, and cried. They were all touching and at the same time heartbreaking. It was from another world; one she was no longer a part of.

After that one time of looking at them, she didn't want to see them again. It reminded her of what she had lost. I never looked at them again, either; the pain of knowing that she would never again be an innocent eleven-year-old was too much for me.

As June edged toward July, I received an e-mail from Hannah's second grade teacher, Marion Tucker. She said, if it wouldn't offend me, she would like to give me her cleaning service for the summer. She and her husband would be away and the service would be cleaning an empty house. It was a wonderful gift, one that lifted a huge burden from my shoulders. I couldn't begin to express my gratitude to her. I accepted, realizing with an enormous sense of relief that when I was home, I didn't need to work all weekend cleaning the house. It also took a burden off Caitlin, who now only had to handle meals, the dog, and general picking up.

As a family, we grudgingly adjusted to living apart. Since Caitlin wasn't able to come to the hospital unless someone gave her a ride, we depended on visitors to bring her. Still, she and Hannah didn't see each other much, relying on phone calls to stay connected. No matter how bad Hannah might be feeling, anytime Caitlin called, she perked up. I often sat listening to Hannah laughing and talking to Caitlin on the phone, only to watch her return to a curled-up ball of misery afterwards. I was truly thankful they had each other.

Caitlin was being a real trouper. I heard from other parents about siblings being angry, acting mean toward the ill child, and acting out. Instead, Caitlin supported Hannah through the hair loss and made her feel okay about herself. She even coveted Hannah's many hats because they were so stylish and cute, making them even more important to Hannah. Whenever Caitlin was at the hospital, I don't think there was more than a foot of distance between them the whole time. She was one of the only people Hannah would let sit on her bed.

Even though we weren't seeing each other, except for quick hugs as one of us arrived and the other departed, Mike and I gave each other a lot of support. We had very different roles in Hannah's care. He was the fun person who read, watched movies, played games, and generally relaxed on the weekends. I was the slave driver, insisting on hospital routines, clean laundry, and regular mealtimes during the week. Throughout our marriage, we had often joked about how well matched we were since we complemented each other's strengths. Of course we were both an amalgam of these two styles and could switch roles if need be. Now that I had discovered cheap phone cards, we talked several times a day, needing to at least hear each other's voices.

For the upcoming weekend at home, I promised myself I wasn't going to worry about anything more than getting some rest, enjoying Caitlin, and doing a few essential errands. I still slept poorly at the hospital, and even though I slept well when I was home, I was always tired. My early morning walks helped some, but being vigilant twenty-four hours a day was exhausting. I put pressure on myself to be strong and cheerful for Hannah. I also felt a need to be professional around the nursing and medical staffs. *They* weren't imposing that on me, *I* was. We had only been at this for a month and I was trying to maintain a sense of perspective, but frequently that was beyond my strength.

On Saturday morning, I slept late and did some minor household chores. Caitlin had been invited to go to the beach with school friends. I was happy she could have some fun while I lazed about. Hoping I could fall asleep in front of the TV, I lay down on the upstairs sofa and thought about how exhausted I felt. Could I keep going at this pace with no idea of how long it would take? There was very little respite from the constant demands of treatment at the hospital. Even when I was home, I wasn't able to relax mentally and let go of my fears.

The task of getting Hannah through this seemed to stretch endlessly into the future, that is, if she even survived. The uncertainty about the possible success of treatment was draining. When would we know how this turned out and how would we know it was over? What if it was never really over? I tried to remind myself that fatigue and fear were the major players in this darkness, but doubts about keeping up with the demands still plagued every waking moment. Today was a day of dark, bleak thoughts. *Wouldn't it be easier, if she wasn't going to make it, to have it happen sooner rather than later?* Immediately, guilt hit hard. Would I lose her as punishment for such a thought? My insides clenched with fear.

Trying to take my mind off my morbid thoughts, I flipped through the TV channels seeking something by which to snooze. I saw that the movie *Terms of Endearment* was on again. It had been on the previous Saturday and Sunday as well as the week before that. I had seen it several times already and knew that it was a tear-jerker, but in the past, when I had watched it, I had no inkling that losing a daughter to cancer could ever be a possibility. So, even though it was very touching, the situation hadn't felt real.

Still wondering why this movie seemed to be on every time I turned on the TV, I gave in and decided to leave it on. I began to follow the story at the point where Emma had just been diagnosed with cancer. I faded in and out of sleep as the characters struggled with their relationships and the meaning of Emma's dying, but came fully awake as Emma was lying in bed in the hospital near the end of her life. Flap, her husband, sat dozing in a chair and Aurora, her mother, sat stiffly across the room from her daughter. *How unreal is that?* What mother would not want to just hold her in her arms, or at the very least, hold her hand? Now I was totally caught up in the movie.

As the next scene unfolded, Emma slowly opened her eyes, focused on her husband asleep in his chair and slowly scanned toward Aurora. They made eye contact. Emma tried to smile. Barely able to lift her hand, she moved her fingers in a feeble wave of parting and then grimaced slightly, closed her eyes, and died. Without moving toward Emma, Aurora gasped and put her hand to her mouth. She stood up, unsteady on her feet, and ran out into the hall calling for the nurse. Aurora stood in the doorway watching the nurse check Emma. The nurse straightened up and shook her head letting Aurora know that Emma really was gone. Aurora's face crumpled as the harsh reality of her loss registered. She walked over to Flap's chair and shook him awake to let him know Emma was dead. Somewhat confused from sleep, he didn't seem to comprehend what had happened.

Aurora grabbed Flap's shoulders and hugged him tightly as she said, "I was wrong. I thought I would be relieved when this was over, because it has been so hard. But this is the hardest thing there is."

Now I knew why this movie had been offered to me over and over again. I needed to hear this. I sat crying, acutely aware of what losing Hannah would mean. I had vowed to do all that it took to help her survive, but with increasing fatigue and stress in the last couple of weeks, I had lost sight of my resolve. This movie reminded me of what I already knew: losing a child would be devastating; I had regained my sense of purpose. No matter how hard this was, the alternative was untenable.

As I sat sifting through my emotions, I had an insight about how I had been handling what had happened thus far. This battle with cancer was an endurance race, not a short sprint. There was no end date to be considered. Each day, every hour was an end in itself. This struggle was no-holds-barred, no regrets, everything left on the field. There was nothing to lose in giving it our all. I realized again how much I needed to let others do; my job was to be Hannah's mom, using love, encouragement, and all of the nursing skills I had to overcome what we were facing. In the end, no matter what happened, I would at least know I had done everything I could to help her win her fight against cancer.

The lack of energy and pervasive sadness I had been feeling was replaced with a new awareness; I could do this no matter what it took. It energized me. I needed to focus on staying fit, making certain I ate healthy, and took time for daily meditation. I needed to see this as a marathon for which I trained each day. If I was able to reframe how I looked at it, I hoped I could keep pace with the effort required. It wouldn't be easy and there would definitely be days when fear, stress, and the constant demands of Hannah's needs would be hard to cope with, but now I finally understood that the alternative was something I could never make peace with.

On Monday morning, with my renewed resolve in place, I packed the car and put my bike in the back along with my helmet and riding gear. Even though I had been walking almost every day, riding would give me a more intense workout. I didn't want to ride in city traffic, but if I started out at the time I usually took my walk, around 5 A.M., I could be back before the traffic became really bad. As long as Hannah was okay and still asleep, it would be easy to get away and have that time for myself. It also gave me something to look forward to each day.

After that, when I stepped out of the hospital each morning, I gratefully breathed in the smell of the ocean, summer flowers, and trees. Once I was on my bike, I flew down the steep hill of the Western Promenade toward the harbor with my spirits soaring. Even with the knowledge that my return to the world of childhood cancer would require standing on the pedals with my legs burning while I climbed back up the hill, that moment of running free kept me going.

Chapter 14
GET-OUT-OF-JAIL-FREE COUNT

Absolute neutrophil count (ANC): the number of circulating neutrophils (infection-fighting cells) in a white blood count.
Test used to determine the ability to fight off infections (<500 indicating high risk) in those receiving chemotherapy.

Our hospital routine depended on how Hannah was feeling. She was still very sick compared to any normal person, and could move from stable to dangerously ill in a matter of minutes. If she was doing okay, she could go to the playroom, watch movies, or even go out on pass, as long as her counts were okay. Decisions about what kind of day it was going to be were often determined on morning medical rounds. When there was good news, the day was a little more relaxed. It was always a relief when we received the official okay for the day; not that this was any guarantee that there wouldn't be a problem five minutes later. At least for that brief moment, we were allowed the illusion that all was going according to plan.

Like every other cancer patient parent, waiting for the daily ANC results, which were announced on rounds, had become my new preoccupation. The whole "rounding" process started before 7 A.M. each day with the medical student assigned to us. She had Hannah as a primary learning responsibility and was the first to examine her and check on how her night had been, but wasn't approved to provide us with any of the results. Her visit tended to be a more informal interaction with mostly a twenty-four-hour history focus and an examination of heart, lungs, skin, eyes, and mouth.

We then awaited the arrival of the full pediatric medical team. First the pediatric residents, interns, and medical students arrived in our room to examine Hannah, at which time our medical student presented the information she had gleaned for the approval of the resident with whom she was training. Then they would all take turns examining Hannah and discuss her case and progress, but they couldn't give us any results either.

The final rounding group was the covering MCCP oncologist and the Nurse Practitioner, both of whom again examined Hannah. From them we received the important information and test results as they discussed where we were on the treatment road map. We were told of any plans for transfusions or further testing, and then our turn was over as they moved on to the next patient. We didn't do anything else except clean up or shower until rounds were completed. Being away from your room when the doctors were rounding could lose you your place in the queue and an even longer wait for information.

I found myself thinking about how naïve I had been when, as a nurse, I had made rounds. While I had been empathetic and had done my best to support and reassure patients, being on the other side of the bed told me no health care professional has any idea what this side feels like. Even the ability to speak the language of medicine did nothing to allay my anxiety about what was happening in treatment.

Since rounds were on a tight schedule, information was given quickly and there wasn't always time for lengthy discussion or questions. I tried very hard to be just Hannah's mom and not let the staff assume I knew things because of my background. We were fortunate to have the MCCP Nurse Practitioner and the nursing staff. They had a wealth of information and knowledge, and were willing to quest for answers from the medical staff. I now fully understood how the next step in the protocol, which seemed routine to staff but was new to patients and family, was sometimes a shock. Even though a specific part of the treatment was listed on the road map, it didn't become real until it was actually a part of care. So the announcement that Hannah would be receiving GCSF shots (granulocyte-colony stimulating factor), also known as G shots, came unexpectedly.

This day, we had been told on rounds that Hannah's ANC was below 100, meaning her counts were the lowest they were likely to be. Each round of chemotherapy had the same objective: destroy all of her bone marrow in hopes of also destroying all of the abnormal leukemia cells. Since bone marrow is made up of blood-forming stem cells, lymphoid tissue, fat cells, and other tissues that aid in the production of blood, bringing her bone marrow back to a healthy level meant stimulating it to resume producing white blood cells. Transfusions took care of platelets and red blood cells, but the GCSF would be needed for white blood cell production.

The theory was that between rounds of chemotherapy, her blood counts would return to normal and her body would only produce healthy cells. For fear of missing some abnormal myeloid cells, multiple rounds of chemo were needed. In each successive round, the bone marrow would be destroyed and rebuilt. Blood counts, specifically the ANC, were the markers in Hannah's progress. The GCSF shots were a key part of the return to normal blood cell levels. Each patient was unique, so no one could say how long it would take---and that determined how long we would have to stay in the hospital in isolation.

I knew what GCSF was, but I had never administered the drug. Kristen, our nurse, came in after rounds to tell us about starting the shots. I had heard talk around the unit about G shots and how much they hurt. Many children had to be held down because they fought so hard not to have them. The skin could be numbed, but the medication itself burned for several minutes after the injection. She wanted us to have a chance to prepare. "Hannah, I'm going to put the EMLA cream on now and then I'll be back in about 15 minutes to give you the shot," Kristen said.

Hannah scowled, but nodded.

As we waited for the spot on her thigh to get numb, I said, "Let's watch a movie. It'll take your mind off the shot."

I sat next to her on the bed and snuggled her tight as we tried to focus on the movie she was watching.

Too soon Kristen returned with the syringe.

"Are you ready Hannah?"

"Not really, but I guess I have to, right?" Hannah said.

Kristen nodded and quickly gave her the shot.

Hannah started to shake and cry yelling, "It hurts! It burns! Mom, make it stop!"

I grabbed her iced water bottle from the bed tray and held it against her leg. As the cold seeped in, she stopped shaking and crying. The medical part of my brain wanted her to have the shots for what they represented in helping her body recover, but the mom part of me wanted to cry with her.

Hannah and I talked about how the ice had helped, so the next day we had the ice ready for when the second injection was finished. She still cried, but the burning went away more quickly. By the third day, Hannah asked if she could have the ice ahead of time to numb her leg before they gave the injection. It worked really well.

She let all of her nurses know she felt this should be the way it was given to all children. She told them if they had the ice first and never learned about how much it hurt, they wouldn't be so afraid. We discovered an additional benefit to this technique: she didn't have as many bruises on her legs from the injection sites, and many of the sites showed no bruising at all. Hannah even reached the point later on of giving her own injections; they were never any picnic, just another task necessary for recovery.

Hannah's counts were climbing and I was excited. Often conversations with other families in treatment included sadly or proudly announcing one's ANC number. If it was high enough, it was celebrated as a minor victory. As strange as it may sound, it felt like the equivalent of winning an all-expenses-paid vacation. The fact the vacation was to one's own home to sleep in one's own bed and be able to cook meals, have privacy, and just be in one place as a family made it unique.

At the rate we were going, there was a chance we would be out of the hospital in a day or two, in time for the Fourth of July holiday. Unfortunately, our hopes were not to be realized. July 1st marks the beginning of the residency and internship year for all of the medical personnel in training. I forgot to tell Mike about it when I went home that weekend.

One of the new residents decided on Sunday night that Hannah's blood pressure was too low. It wasn't any different than it usually was, but we had the misfortune of having a float nurse who wasn't familiar with Hannah and this resident who also wasn't knowledgeable about her case. Perhaps neither of them could read a chart very well because her BP certainly wasn't significantly lower than was normal for her. He decided, without checking with the oncologist on call, to infuse 500 milliliters of normal saline. Her blood pressure certainly came up, but now her blood counts had been changed, and our lives were governed by what her counts showed.

I found out about it when I came in on Monday morning. The consequences of this became clear on rounds. Because of the dilution, her ANC had dropped, and with it our chance to go home in a few days. I was angry and let Dr. Hurwitz know. He addressed the issue, but it didn't change the result. It was another reminder about how crucial being constantly vigilant was; we needed to question *everything* being done to Hannah. This incident reinforced my feeling that any hospitalized patient in the complicated world of medical care today needs an advocate present at all times.

Teaching hospitals with house staff provide a wonderful way to train new doctors, but having worked in Boston hospitals with interns and residents, I had my own prejudices. Mike would have had no way of knowing he needed to insist that this resident speak with the oncologist on call. We learned a valuable lesson and now neither of us was afraid to ask "why" before anything new or out of the ordinary was done.

Hannah was very disappointed. She had been looking forward to attending our large community fireworks celebration. It was held on the university campus, and people from our town and many surrounding towns always attended. We usually saw friends with whom we didn't have regular contact. Instead, we all sat looking out the window of the teen room. We discovered fireworks were not nearly as interesting if you couldn't hear the sound along with the display. They were beautiful, but disappointing. It drove home one more lesson about what living in the hospital did to daily life. We could see sunshine, thunderstorms, rainbows, and rich foliage outside our window, but like the fireworks, there was no sound, no smell, and none of the splendor of summer days.

Chapter 15
GOOD NEWS AND BAD NEWS

Remission: slowing of disease, lessening of symptoms,
or their temporary reduction or disappearance.

Almost before I got used to sleeping in my own bed again, another six days at home had passed. We were scheduled for a second bone marrow biopsy and aspiration on July 11th that would tell us if the first round of chemotherapy had put Hannah into remission.

We arrived at 7:30 A.M. at the ASU (Ambulatory Surgery Unit) at MMC, where the procedure would be done, to find a line at the registration desk. Before I stood in line, I found a spot for us on one of the soft couches so Hannah could sit down while I checked her in. The place was a bustle of activity with people coming and going. The orange, green, and yellow soft vinyl couches and hard plastic bucket chairs lined up in rows along every wall and in double rows down the center of the room gave it the appearance of a bus station waiting room. Repeated loudspeaker announcements contributed to the image as people were called to various stops on the road to care or treatment.

Once I reached the head of the line, I recited the now familiar insurance and billing information litany and signed consent forms for both anesthesia and the bone marrow biopsy. I was glad I had found us seats first, as fifteen minutes later an open seat came at a premium. We snuggled together on one end of our couch and read our books while we waited for Hannah's name to be called.

Despite my love of people-watching, I was learning, in these situations, not to be too interested in the stories of those around us. Some people were clearly suffering and uncomfortable, some in wheelchairs and others on crutches, and despite some obvious maladies, I didn't really want to know anything about them. I didn't work here and wasn't in a position to do anything to help anyone but Hannah. She whispered to me asking questions about some of the people who came and went. I told her that we could only imagine and hope that they could be helped.

I wondered what any of them thought of her. She had been feeling fine at home and looked good. The only giveaway to her condition was her bald head, which was covered by her blue flowered hat, so her hair loss wasn't obvious to anyone but us. I tried not to obsess about the importance of today's results. If the first round of chemotherapy had been successful, her bone marrow biopsy would show normal blood cells and no blast cells. Since she seemed to have recovered from the first round so well, I could only hope our news would be good.

I thought about all we had been through in the last seven weeks. It was hard to believe that the presence of her central line, central line dressing changes, blood draws and treatments which had been very scary, all now seemed quite commonplace. I continued to be amazed at her ability to cope with all she faced every day. She was cooperative and responsible about all of the preventive measures required each day to keep her mouth and GI tract healthy. While it may have helped that I had given her control over scheduling things that were not time-sensitive, she never argued or fought with me about what had to be done. She was comfortable, with some help, flushing her central line ports and setting up the sterile field for her dressing changes. She took her own temperature each morning, completed her mouth care, and took her medications without question. Some days I didn't know which one of us was supporting and which one needed the support. I hoped that she was able to take strength from me, because I certainly found my spirits bolstered by her positive and cheerful attitude.

Now, she was totally at ease about having another surgery. Being NPO (nothing by mouth) wasn't a big deal anymore, and she knew what it felt like to have anesthesia. She knew she might not feel well immediately afterward, but that she would be okay later. This morning in the car, she had talked again about how anesthesia felt.

"Last time they did this I felt like I was in a different world. Remember, you said you always felt that way too," she said.

"Yeah, that's always strange. For me it was always so vivid, I felt I must live there," I said.

"When they were trying to wake me up after, it was like it had only been a minute or two and I really wanted to stay in that other world. It was a great place."

"I'll bet it was! Maybe that's why you're supposed to think pleasant thoughts before they put the medication in. Maybe it helps you get to the great place faster."

"Um, I don't know. Could be," she said.

I thought about this conversation and smiled as I snuggled her a little tighter.

Finally, her name was called and we were taken to the pre-op area. To our delight and surprise, the same anesthesiologist that did her first bone marrow biopsy was doing the anesthesia. Hannah was happy to see him and had a couple of jokes for him. They chatted as he completed his exam and then he said he would see her inside.

There weren't any "older kid" books in this part of the pediatric area, so we read some Dr. Seuss books together. I sat in the rocking chair reading aloud while Hannah sat cross-legged on the stretcher. We laughed together over these books we hadn't read since she was little. Ah, that world of innocence and small worries seemed so wonderful; I wished we could magically go back.

I watched Hannah being wheeled into the OR and waved from behind a watery smile. It would be at least an hour before she would be in recovery. I walked to the coffee shop with my book to have a cup of tea, but got worried after just a few minutes and quickly walked back to the ASU in case they needed to find me.

Perhaps it was wishful thinking, but I felt that the first round had destroyed the cancer. Even if she was in remission, I knew I didn't have the courage to say to the oncologists, "She's cured. We should leave well enough alone and just keep checking her each week for blast cells." If some cancer was still there and we didn't continue treatment, I knew I wouldn't forgive myself. Still, part of me wanted to say that sentence and be done.

Lost in my reverie, I didn't realize my name was being called. When I finally heard it, I quickly grabbed my things and hurried to the desk.

The clerk pointed to a nurse and said, "They're ready for you in recovery."

I scanned the nurse's face for any signs of problems and breathed a sigh of relief as she said, "Hannah did very well and is starting to wake up. She's in the same cubicle. As soon as she's taking fluids and steady on her feet, you can take her home."

"Thanks."

Hannah was sleeping peacefully. I whispered a silent "thank you" and breathed a sigh of relief. Leaning over, I gave her a big hug and a kiss.

She hugged me back and sleepily said, "Hi, Mom."

"I'm glad to see you woke up cheerful, big bug."

She smiled as she drifted back to sleep.

At home again, she was happy to be sleeping in her own bed and didn't seem to care about when we would get results. The two days until they came seemed to take forever for me, but there was good news. She was in remission! I was relieved and excited, but depressingly, that meant she would start the second round of chemotherapy on July 17th.

All our preparations for a return to the hospital were complete, and I hoped to spend the two days we had left at home relaxing. I was downstairs doing paper work when I heard Hannah shouting.

"Mom! Mom! Come here!"

I took the stairs two at a time and ran to her room.

"What? What's the matter?"

"There's blood in my bed!"

I climbed onto her upper bunk and pulled her shirt up searching for the central line port clamps. Thankfully, they were still closed. I checked her over and found nothing else.

"Does anything hurt?" I asked.

"Not really; I had some stomach cramps during the night," she said.

I was shocked; her body was following its own schedule. How, under these conditions, had she started her menses? Could her body be doing something so normal for the first time when she had just been through a round of chemotherapy? Could this really mean she was cured? We could only hope!

Needless to say, I had envisioned this moment very differently; a celebration, special lunch, new outfit, or any number of other ways to make her feel special. My excitement died immediately. We were about to start chemo again. Once her platelets went down, bleeding would be a major problem. While she took a shower, I called MCCP to see if this changed their plans for admission. It didn't. The only change they would make was in the order of the chemotherapy agents, not the overall plan. Our admission would go on as scheduled.

Chapter 16
HURDLES

*Complication: a disease or problem that arises in addition
to the initial condition or during a surgical operation.*

From the start, things did not go well. All of the regular rooms designated for patients with cancer were full, and in addition, there was a chance Hannah had been exposed to Fifth's Disease (a viral infection which causes minimal problems in most children). We hoped it wouldn't make Hannah very sick even if she did have it. The symptoms were self-limiting and mild, much like a cold with a low-grade fever and a rash that gave kids a "slapped cheeks" appearance. Hannah had a bit of a snuffle and her cheeks were redder than usual, but otherwise she felt fine.

We were put into one of the negative-pressure rooms which functions the opposite of the positive-pressure rooms by not letting any air from the room out into the hall. Since we were only supposed to be here for five days as they started round two, I wasn't particularly concerned. As long as she stayed in the room, she wasn't a risk to anyone else.

The treatment map was altered to exclude the Danorubicin, which caused a faster decrease in platelets. Since her platelets were still okay now, the oncologists decided to wait until she was home from this hospitalization to see a gynecologist for cycle suppression. I was feeling very confident that this hospital stay would be very straightforward. We had come in on Thursday and she was scheduled to be discharged on Tuesday, so I hadn't bothered to bring much with us. Mike would stay the weekend and then I would come on Sunday night for the last couple of days.

Our best laid plans, of course, were not to be. During the weekend, Hannah developed a fever that exceeded their protocol limit of 100.4F. They drew blood cultures looking for possible sources of infection. I was convinced this was probably the Fifth's Disease and would be gone in a day or two. Her counts were good, so even if it weren't viral, she would still have a chance of fighting a bacterial infection.

All my confidence about sailing through this round vanished with the results of the blood cultures during Monday morning's medical rounds. Hannah's central line was infected. This wasn't news I wanted or expected to hear. We discussed the choices. I hoped they could just give her antibiotics through her central line and kill off whatever germs were in there. Their past experience with central lines dictated the protocol. Bacteria could be hiding in and around the cuff, which kept the central line in place, where the antibiotics might not kill them. They had no choice but to remove it; she was immediately put on the OR schedule for later in the day.

In the meantime she was started on antibiotics. Since they needed some type of intravenous line while the infection was being treated, it was decided that a PICC line (a long intravenous line which is inserted into a vein in the arm and then threaded into the vena cava in the chest) would be inserted. It would serve as a temporary replacement for a central line until the infection was cleared. These lines lasted longer than peripheral IVs, and were stable and safe for medications and blood transfusions which would irritate peripheral veins. After a lengthy discussion between Dr. Hamilton and the pediatric surgeon, they decided to use a modified PICC line. It would be shorter than usual since they only needed it for a few days until she had clean blood cultures and could have another central line put in.

Trips to the OR were becoming a habit I didn't like, but we were assured this would be quick. I went to the cafeteria for lunch thinking that by the time I was done eating, they should be calling me to go down to the recovery room.

When I got back to the unit, they hadn't yet had a call, so I put the room in order and sat down to wait. After an hour passed, I walked out to the nurse's station again to inquire if they had heard anything. There was some discussion and then the nurse told me that Hannah should be in recovery soon. I felt a little disquieted by the fact that this seemed to be taking a lot longer than anticipated, but assumed there could have been a delay in getting started.

Another hour passed; now I was really worried. The nurses told me the surgeon should be coming up to talk with me shortly. In fact, a few minutes later Dr. Hamilton came in to tell me there had been a problem with the insertion of the PICC line. Instead of using a cut-down version, they had attempted to insert a full-length PICC line. Unfortunately, Hannah's vein had gone into spasm and they were unable to advance it.

Since they couldn't have a large loop of the IV line on the outside of her body, they needed to remove it, and that was where the real trouble lay. Hannah's vein had clamped down around the line and now they could neither advance nor remove it.

Once again, I rushed through the recovery room doors. I looked toward the pediatric area, but it was dark. On the far side of the room, I saw the individually lit stretchers of the eight remaining postoperative patients of the day. It was quiet compared to the usual level of noise, and when I finally spotted Hannah, she looked bulky under the sheet covering her. They had put the "bear hugger" (warming blanket that circulates heated air) on her. Just her left arm with loops of the ill-fated PICC line was showing, and I could see tear stains on her cheeks. The nurse was bathing her arm in warmed saline attempting to get the vein to relax.

"Mom's here. Are you in pain, sweet girl?"

"No, I'm hot. They won't take this blanket thing off of me."

Because she had spent a long time on the operating table, her temperature had dipped very low and now they needed to warm her. She kept trying to get her legs out from under it and the nurse kept putting them back.

"What's her temperature?" I asked.

"She is still only 35.9C [normal is 37C] and we really want to return her temperature to a more normal range before we take her upstairs. They also need to remove the PICC line. I know it really hurts since her vein is still in spasm, but the warm soaks should decrease that," the nurse said.

I looked at Hannah.

"They need to get the line out of your arm and then you can rest a while longer before you go back upstairs," I said. "I know you feel hot, but your body hasn't warmed up enough yet. As soon as your temperature is more normal they'll take the blanket off."

She closed her eyes and nodded. Later she told me that she had worked really hard in her half-awake state to get one of her feet out from under the warming blanket and just when she felt the cool relief of success, the nurse noticed and said, "Oops, one little foot escaped. We can't have that if you're going to warm up." Hannah said that she thought to herself, *Foiled again, just when I thought I had escaped*. At least later she was able laugh instead of cry.

Each attempt at removal of the line had been very painful. As I stood there rubbing her shoulder and holding her hand, the pediatric surgeon came to check on her, apologize, and explain to me what had happened. While we were talking, the nurse pulled the catheter a little further out of her arm. Hannah shrieked. Most of the other patients in the recovery room sat up wondering what had happened. I held Hannah while the rest of the catheter was removed, she continued to writhe in pain until the pain medication took effect and she fell asleep again.

The pediatric surgeon patted my back and Hannah's leg as he apologized again. I waited until he left and then put my head down on the bed rail and cried. What else would go wrong? This had been a terrible few days.

When Hannah woke up, the nurse told her that all of the other nurses were grateful to her for waking up several of the patients that they had been trying to rouse from anesthesia. Hannah was able to laugh a little and we joked about getting her a job in the recovery room waking up patients. She wasn't happy about the PICC line fiasco, but now that it was over, she could let it go. Once again her resilience and humor helped her get through a tough situation. I needed to learn from this child; my own sense of humor had gone south some hours before and all I felt was anger and frustration with no outlet. I knew unexpected things happened in patient care; I just didn't want them happening to her.

Finally, Hannah was back in her room asleep. I lay on the parent couch trying to find sleep, worried about what else might go wrong. My earlier optimism was gone and I was rapidly learning more about what a powerful enemy infection was.

The days of waiting for the infection to clear were frustrating. The peripheral lines didn't last long, as they became inflamed or stopped working because the antibiotics and blood transfusions caused irritation. The biggest concern was a phlebitis (inflammation of a vein) which could cause additional problems. Showering was difficult and she was back to wearing hospital gowns with their snap sleeves to avoid entanglement with IV lines. The worst part was having blood drawn once a day (sometimes more) through the veins in her hands and arms. She had lots of bruises and was sporting hot packs to decrease the soreness and inflammation of veins in both arms.

This second round of chemotherapy felt as if we were spiraling into an ever-deepening morass. If we were making any progress, it wasn't evident. It now felt as if we had sailed through the first round. Logically, I remembered terrible days during our first two hospitalizations, but this seemed worse. It was hard to remember that the high of one day could easily be succeeded by a terrible low the next, and vice versa.

Finally, at the end of the week we had good news: the blood cultures had come back negative. Perhaps things would be better now that she would have a new central line, the suppression therapy for her menses would keep the bleeding risks down, and she would finally start to feel better.

Now that things began to settle down medically, we faced insurance worries again. Although Mike's company's situation seemed okay at the moment, there were rumors of buy outs or closure. Liz, our social worker, had helped me complete the paperwork for application to Katie Beckett Funds. This was a state Medicaid program, a "Healthy Kids Gold" initiative to provide insurance coverage for children with a disability who were uninsured or might become uninsured while in the midst of a severe illness.

The application required an in-person interview. Before I went back to the hospital on the Monday, I drove to the welfare office. Nothing in the building was clearly marked, and after several false starts, I finally found the correct office. Inside, in the glare of neon lights, a dejected-looking group of people sat on plastic chairs waiting their turns. The receptionist was behind a bullet-proof glass window with an intercom for communication. I gave my name and additional forms were slid into the tray under the window. I joined those on the hard plastic chairs to complete more paperwork. It was difficult to make sense of the wording, which included barely intelligible fine print. I wondered how people who needed these services, but were poorly educated, found their way through the system. I had a master's degree and I felt as if these forms were written in a foreign language.

When I was finally shown into a claustrophobic cubicle masquerading as an interview room, I could feel the caseworker's hostility. She barely made eye contact as she wrote notes on each form. She questioned me at length on why I was applying for this, but then seemed to ignore my answers. Her tone of voice implied that I was trying to get something undeserved or was taking advantage of the poor tax payer who was "footing the bill." I felt guilty for even having this need by the time the interview was over. How depressing it must be for those who had to do this regularly. I accepted the need to jump through the hoops because if we lost insurance at any time, we needed this as back up. Most of the other people here needed it just to help their kids get *any* medical care.

The mounting cost of treatment was not something over which we had any control, but each time I reviewed the itemized bills for Hannah's care, I felt sick to my stomach. It reminded me of something I had read about our broken health care payment system: "We are all just one major illness away from bankruptcy". We weren't even halfway through what was planned as treatment and our costs were in the hundreds of thousands of dollars.

Hannah had been back to the OR for placement of a new central line. Thankfully, nothing had gone wrong with that, so far. We moved into one of the regular rooms in the cancer treatment section for the second part of this second round of chemo. I thought we were back on track as we meticulously followed our prevention protocols for her eyes, mouth and skin, but now Hannah had developed a "minor" cold. Even though it was initially a viral infection, it had lingered and settled in her sinuses. Now her tear ducts were blocked, her eyes were light-sensitive, and she had a sinus infection. I worried all weekend at home about it worsening.

The phone woke me around two o'clock Monday morning. Late-night phone calls did not bode well, and my mind raced through all kinds of bad thoughts in the few seconds it took me to answer. It was Mike.

"Is Hannah okay?" I blurted out.

"She still has her sinus infection and her eyes continue to hurt, but that isn't why I called you. The pediatric resident wants to give her morphine because the sinus pain hasn't gotten better," Mike said. "I told him he had to talk with you since our last resident experience wasn't great."

"Okay, sure," I said.

A voice on the other end of the line said, "I'm the resident on call and we don't want to give Hannah any more acetaminophen for pain because she's had quite a lot today."

"Has she been complaining of pain?" I asked.

"No," he replied. "The nurse was taking vital signs and noted that Hannah still has pain."

"So, let me get this straight," I said. "She was sound asleep and not being kept awake by the pain, but after they awakened her for her vital signs and eye drops, she complained of pain."

"Yes," he answered.

"You know that she had a difficult time with morphine before. It gave her bad stomach cramps and diarrhea."

"No, I didn't know that," he said.

"Can we use something in between, like codeine, if she can't sleep?"

"Yeah, I suppose we can," he replied.

Mike was glad he had called after I relayed my conversation with the resident. Knowing that Mike would keep an eye on Hannah until I arrived, I thought I would be able to go back to sleep, but my mind wouldn't shut down. Cancer was an intimidating diagnosis, but the secondary infections were just as scary. I was willing to do whatever protocol demanded in the chemotherapy treatment, but that didn't affect these problems.

Since I couldn't sleep, I decided to go in early to spend a little time with Mike. A couple of thoughts had kept coming up since Mike's call. I was so intimidated by the word cancer that I hadn't been able to think about other approaches, like some complementary therapies, which might help her. I didn't know how the oncologists would feel about it, but I knew I could help her with the sinus infection, and possibly with her eyes as well.

I shared with Mike what I proposed to do and he agreed it wouldn't hurt to try. Hannah was awake and feeling terrible, so I told her that I had decided to try some of our other methods for helping her get rid of her cold and sinus problems. I kept the room dark and gave her a pair of sunglasses for her eyes so they wouldn't be so painful. I filled a basin with very hot water and put a towel over her head so that she could breathe steam to loosen some of the congestion. I then did Cranial Sacral Therapy (CST) and Foot Reflexology to help her sinuses drain and clear her clogged tears ducts. Because she had felt so bad, she hadn't been drinking as much as she needed to, so I pushed her to drink a lot more. After we finished, she got cleaned up and then slept comfortably for a while.

After rounds, an ENT (Ear, Nose and Throat) specialist came to examine Hannah. The pediatric staff and oncologists were discussing the possibility of starting her on an antibiotic that required permission from the CDC to use, or taking her to the OR to clean out her sinuses--or both. Since these options were less than ideal, I decided to speak frankly with the ENT doctor about trying the alternative approaches first. To my surprise, he agreed. He said that if there was any other way to help with this problem, he was okay with it; he didn't relish taking a patient with a compromised immune system to surgery unless there was no other choice. He said anything that would help her clear her sinuses on her own was definitely preferable, and he would be happy to check back the next day to see how she was progressing. I was relieved to have such an open response to complementary therapies.

Thrilled to have found something more I could do for her, I continued the treatments throughout the day, and by evening her sinuses were clearing and her tear ducts weren't blocked anymore. The next day, she didn't need the sunglasses, but wore them because they were cool. The chemotherapy might be essential to her survival in terms of the cancer, but there were other choices for the secondary complications.

Later in the week, Dr. Hurwitz asked me about what I had done, so I explained what the therapies were. He offered to schedule a consult with a doctor who was trained in both Western and Chinese medicine. He added that astragalus, an immune booster, seemed to decrease the number of fevers in their patients. It was very reassuring to learn that the oncologists were open to more than just one approach to patient problems.

Chapter 17
STAGNATION

Doldrums: a sluggish state in which no development or improvement occurs. Weather conditions that cause sailing ships to become becalmed.

We had been given a few days at home after the chemotherapy was finished, but when Hannah developed a low-grade fever, we weren't able to stay. Blood cultures didn't show any signs of infection, but now she would be an inpatient until her ANC returned to an infection-fighting level. As long as Hannah felt okay, I was able to relax about being there. We had our routines, and now that Hannah felt completely comfortable with all of the staff and facilities, she came and went seeking out ways to fight boredom.

One of the new distractions we found was following Lance Armstrong's efforts to win a fourth Tour de France. We watched eagerly each day. He was an inspirational hero to follow. He had fought through cancer and afterwards returned to compete in the hardest bike race in the world. He had not only triumphed over his cancer, but was an athlete determined to fulfill his dreams. Hannah and I cheered with each of his triumphs on his way to Paris. We also read his book, *It's Not About the Bike,* out loud together. It gave Hannah a different view of cancer: the only outcomes weren't death or permanent disability.

Still, our most welcome distractions came from having visitors. Arlene, one of the soccer moms on the team, often made the trip with her daughter Emily, and always brought Caitlin along. Hannah's best friend, Ellen Claire, came with her mom, Margery. It was great support for me and gave Hannah someone to be with for at least part of the long days. Having to wear a mask no longer bothered her, so when she didn't have visitors she sought out other kids in the play or teen rooms.

"Mom, I met a new girl in the playroom. She's not sick, but her older sister is."

"Why is her sister here?"

"I think its leukemia, but not like mine."

"Was it ALL [acute lymphocytic leukemia]?"

"Could be," she said.

The girl was Hannah's age and her older sister, Andrea, had in fact just been admitted with ALL. The whole family was spending a lot of time on the unit, and this little girl was bored and looking for someone to play with. I was glad Hannah had found a new friend. I wasn't concerned about Hannah becoming overwhelmed. She would take breaks to come to her room to rest if she became tired, but for the sake of my own mental health, I still tried to keep some distance from other families without being unfriendly.

However, later that week one of the nurses asked me if I would be willing to be introduced to this child's mom, since she had a lot of questions about all that was happening. Even though the type of cancer was different and had another treatment protocol, the effect of a cancer diagnosis on families was similar.

We talked about the unit and all of the available services. Many of the questions she had didn't have answers at this point, and I could only reassure her that the care here was excellent and they would do everything they could to help her daughter. My professional skills and comfort in dealing with families of patients in my care took over for a few minutes. I talked with her and gave support, but it wasn't personal. At the same time, I knew this was my life too, and I suddenly felt like an old hand at the game of cancer treatment. It was very strange to see someone else experiencing the early stages we had been through only a couple of months ago. I recognized the "deer-in-the-headlights" look on their faces and realized our own first experiences seemed a long time ago. We hadn't been doing this that long, but a cancer diagnosis and treatment ages you rapidly in the experience realm. Every test, every procedure, was frightening, and waiting for results was nerve-wracking no matter how much inside knowledge I had---and they had none.

A couple of days later, I had an opportunity to learn something about how Hannah saw her treatment experience, when she interacted with this family. She was sitting on her bed after having her blood drawn. The large door to the hall was open and Hannah saw Andrea sitting in a wheelchair by the nurse's station.

To my surprise, Hannah called out to her, "Where are you going?"

She answered, "Uh, I think X-ray."

"Oh, X-ray isn't bad. Nothing they do is painful and the people are really nice and funny," Hannah said.

I was surprised that Hannah felt comfortable initiating a conversation with an older teenager, but then my jaw actually dropped when she lifted off her hat and displayed her very bald head.

"It's not so bad and it grows back when you're done," Hannah said.

The girl smiled shyly and said, "Thank you."

After she was wheeled away, I said, "That was a really nice thing to do, Hannah. Did you know she was worried about her hair?"

"Yeah, her sister said she loves her long black hair and was crying about it falling out."

"Well, I'm sure it made her feel a little better seeing that you're okay with losing your hair. Maybe she won't be so worried about it."

"It really is okay, Mom. I know my hair will grow back eventually."

I gave her a big hug and asked permission to kiss her beautiful, bald head. It was so soft and smooth that I loved touching and kissing it. Today she let me. Then I walked away so that she wouldn't see my tears and think I was upset. I wasn't. I was just so proud of my wonderful daughter with her generous and loving soul.

That Friday, the child and her family were discharged after their initial stage of treatment. Other than to appreciate Hannah and her sensitivity, I didn't think much more about the experience.

I had always seen hospital rooms as functional spaces, but living in one for an extended period of time required a new approach. If we were stuck here, I wanted to make Hannah's room more personal. The mother of an older child who needed to be in isolation for several weeks showed us the Hawaiian-themed room she had created. Hannah thought decorating would be fun and wanted a marine theme. I brought from home two yards of deep blue fabric printed with whales and dolphins for covering the hallway window; it was decorative and blocked out light at night.

Hannah's friend Eileen had given her a three-foot-long, neon green alligator with purple trim. She named him Larry and frequently used him to terrorize unsuspecting night nurses by having his head sticking out of the covers when they came to take vital signs. During the day, he lived at the foot of her bed.

She had a large, well-loved bear from her friend Lia, and one of the evening nurses had given her a big, soft Gund dolphin. She also had Lovey and Sealy, her white seal. All of these animals lived around her pillow to keep her company during the day and be available for snuggling when she was having a bad time. Friends had sent her glow-in-the-dark reusable plastic stick-on pictures of tropical fish, which we used to decorate her door and the walls in front of her bed. I found a fish-shaped wind chime, and we hung it on the curtain track so that it chimed anytime someone opened the door or moved the curtains. Later I found, in the Old Port section of Portland, a beautiful kite with a purple background and three dolphins leaping together in a center circle. It looked beautiful on the ceiling above her bed.

In the family area on the unit, there were quilts, afghans, and knitted hats donated by the "grandmas" who gave gifts to the pediatric unit. Hannah picked out a couple of hats to wear and two different blankets for her bed. The wife of one of the nurses had been Hannah's elementary school music teacher. She had made a beautiful quilt which he brought in for Hannah. It was one of her favorites and stayed on her bed most of the time. All of these wonderful touches didn't keep it from being a hospital room, lessen the boredom or make it less difficult to be there, but it did feel as if we were being proactive in decreasing some of the potential for "hospitalitis".

As the food issue continued to be a problem, we tried to be creative in our approaches to solving it. Hannah had definite food cravings, but many of the items available on the hospital menu didn't appeal to her. Our solution to the morning sandwich craving was to cook in the family area on the unit. There was only a microwave oven and a toaster, but I became adept at cooking eggs and turkey bacon in the microwave, topping them with cheese to serve on a toasted English muffin. One or two of these sandwiches became her breakfast and sometimes other meals during the day, as well. The only problem was that suddenly there were lots of children craving bacon, as the aroma was hard to contain. I noticed several other parents cooking bacon; we had started a trend.

Hannah went through various types of cravings as the weeks passed. One day, she had a craving for Mexican food. Not knowing all of the restaurants in the area, I walked to the one that I did know about in the historic Old Port almost three miles away. I trekked down there, bought Mexican food, and hurried back to her room so that it wouldn't be too cold. As she was eating it, one of the nurses came in and asked if I had gone to the Mexican restaurant just below the hospital in the little strip mall. We laughed and decided that at least I had earned what she was eating with my long walk. Now that we knew about the closer place, she and Mike frequently had Mexican food on the weekends, as it was one of his favorite types of food, too.

Her other two cravings were for tortilla chips with Newman's Own salsa and falafel wraps. Hannah later told me it was such an unreal world that she didn't really think much about asking me to go foraging for any foods she craved. Since there wasn't a lot to do, I didn't mind, as long as she wasn't having a bad day. Most other parents played similar roles because the concern was about making certain the child ate and didn't lose weight.

As we entered the fourth week in the hospital and Hannah's counts began to return to an acceptable level with the G shots, it was hard to have to stay. Friends still continued to bring Caitlin to visit whenever they could, but Mike and I only saw each other in passing or talked on the phone. We wanted to be all together again at home.

Hannah wasn't having any complications, so we finally let Liz make arrangements for Mike and me to stay at the Ronald McDonald House. Caitlin spent the night with a friend while we had a lovely dinner together and stayed overnight. It was the only time one of us did not sleep in Hannah's room. Despite my trust in the nursing staff, I had to force myself not to call repeatedly to see if she was okay.

Although it was great to be together, Mike found being around the other people there, who had children with terrible problems, a little depressing. I didn't mind as much. I had become used to closing my awareness to the problems around me that I couldn't do anything about. It was so good just to be able to talk face to face. Of course, we weren't able to stay off the topic of our day-to-day struggles, but we tried hard to talk about other things.

My sanity was still dependent on my morning bike ride and a walk whenever I could find the time. One afternoon as I was leaving for a walk, I saw the father of the teenager Hannah had encouraged not to worry about losing her hair. I was surprised to see him, and asked after his daughter. He began to cry as he told me that Andrea had developed complications and was in the PICU. I was shocked. He explained that her bowel had ruptured due to constipation. She hadn't told her parents about the stomach cramps and how bad she felt because she wanted to go out with friends.

My heart was pounding so hard I felt sick to my stomach. Everyone in cancer treatment was always just one misstep away from a disastrous complication. There wasn't much I could say or do other than offer my sympathy. As I walked I thought, *Thank God Hannah isn't old enough to be out on her own.* I watched her like a hawk for any signs of problems, but I could understand how an older teenager might think. She probably just wanted to go back to being a high school kid who could be with her friends without having to worry about cancer. Life wasn't fair.

When I returned, I found Hannah already knew about the situation. Her friend had been in the playroom. We talked about what had happened and I explained what I knew about this type of complication, reassuring her that this didn't always happen. She seemed sad, but didn't want to talk more about it. I let it go.

Unfortunately, the story didn't end there. A few days later, Hannah's little friend came bursting into our room crying, to tell us that her sister was being taken off life support. Liz was right behind her, but hadn't been able to catch up to her as she ran out of the PICU. Hannah started to cry and could only say how sorry she was. Hannah's counts were very low just then, which placed her at high risk for complications, so she wasn't able to offer more than words. We sat together crying and talking about how sad it was. Andrea was just the first of several children Hannah got to know who later died of their disease or of complications. I had no words of consolation for an eleven-year-old who was finding out that death is a part of life, sometimes even for children.

Chapter 18
A RESERVED GIFT OF CELLS

BMT (Bone Marrow Transplantation): process whereby bone marrow taken from a donor is transplanted into another person who isn't making healthy blood cells.

Except for two days at home the first weekend in August, Hannah had been in the hospital since the middle of July. It had been a long and tedious four weeks. Now that round two was over, I could only hope that we had fulfilled our quota of complications and sadness. Maybe we would be luckier in the next round and have fewer problems, but I wasn't holding my breath.

As we prepared to go home, Dr. Hurwitz came in to discuss the next step in the process. We were scheduled to have a consult at Dana-Farber Cancer Institute in Boston to decide whether Hannah should proceed immediately to bone marrow transplant, since we had Caitlin as her donor. Having not thought beyond the end of round two, the discussion was unsettling and took me by surprise. Logically, it was very reasonable, but I hadn't even considered doing anything but what was planned for here. The problems and fear we knew were more acceptable than the unknown.

Although I knew about bone marrow transplants and generally what was involved, I had many questions and didn't want to feel that a rash decision was being made without full consideration of the consequences. I trusted the MCCP oncologists and believed that they would consider our concerns as a part of the equation, but I didn't know how much it was just assumed, in cancer treatment circles, that she would have a transplant.

The exact statistical odds for a cure from chemotherapy versus transplantation weren't something I knew offhand, but I hoped the final decision would be based on a total picture, including all of the side effects and potential complications. The thought of both my children in the hospital, even if one was helping the other, was scary. Clearly, Caitlin was willing to be Hannah's donor if we went that route, but it would be hard for her. I didn't want to minimize the enormity of the decision and what it would mean to have the burden for "saving Hannah" fall on her shoulders.

We came home on Friday and our appointment in Boston was on Tuesday the 20th. Mike searched the internet to get as much information as he could before we went. I had never worked in a transplant unit, but I knew the effects of destroying all of Hannah's bone marrow with radiation. If she had a transplant of Caitlin's marrow, the stem cells she received would restart Hannah's marrow producing healthy cells. There was no way to know if chemotherapy would have been enough if we elected transplantation with its additional complications.

My thoughts returned to the child who had gone through all of the rounds of chemo and then relapsed a year later. It was very disheartening to think about the possibility that we could complete chemotherapy, be in remission, and still have to do this. While I didn't know if transplantation was the right choice, I kept asking myself whether it wouldn't be better to just go that route since the cure rate was statistically better. I had a running commentary in my head about the pros and cons of each choice when I couldn't sleep during the nights leading up to our appointment. I knew logically that there was no a guarantee either way, but I wanted there to be.

Whenever Hannah didn't feel well or was especially tired, I assumed the worst with the relapse nemesis hovering over my shoulder. Each time she had blood drawn, I had a knot in my stomach from a day or two prior until they called us a day or two later with the results. If Hannah survived, this fear would probably be with me the rest of my life. It all felt like random chance, but for now she was in remission and I had hope.

Boston traffic was heavy as we drove to Dana Farber. I was grateful we had been able to have treatment at Maine Medical Center (MMC), because as much as I loved Boston as a city, driving there on a regular basis was stressful, even if you were doing it for fun. The thought of having to drive an ill child to a clinic or admission to the hospital was nightmarish.

When we finally found the entrance to the parking garage, I realized the parking spaces were underground. Our descent was through a winding maze with a steep gradient and sharp turns. Three or four levels down, we finally spotted a parking space. I tried to keep my own demons about places like this under control while we searched for the correct elevator to take us back to the surface level and daylight. Mike wasn't bothered by it, and Caitlin and Hannah seemed fine as we headed upward, but suffice it to say, I wouldn't have made a very good ore miner.

We were entering a new medical system with the requisite completion of paperwork and insurance forms. While I took care of the bureaucracy, Caitlin, Mike, and Hannah sat in the congested waiting area with other families.

The atmosphere was very different from MCCP. Everyone was very pleasant, but the sheer numbers of people waiting made it seem hectic. Always aware of the infection risk, I worried Hannah was being exposed to some new infectious disease because of the large numbers of young children playing in the area. Her counts were currently high enough to fight an infection, so I resisted the urge to force everyone in the room to cover their mouth and wash their hands.

We were finally ushered into an examination room to meet the Dana Farber transplantation specialists. Dr. Gruinen, the energetic and charming head of the team, popped into the room to explain their role in our treatment decision. She introduced Dr. Thornby, who would be seeing Hannah. I immediately liked him, partly because of his proper British accent, but mostly for his kind, gentle manner and the aura of competence that surrounded him.

Introductions and pleasantries out of the way, Dr. Thornby completed his initial interview and examination.

When he was finished he asked, "Do you really have cancer, Hannah?"

She looked very puzzled and said, "Yes. Why?"

"You look so healthy and vibrant, it's hard to believe what your medical record says," he answered.

We all laughed.

"I just hope she stays that way," I said.

"I hope so too," he said.

"I am really surprised that with only your sister to test from there is a five out of six donor match. Just to be certain, I want to repeat the HLA testing for both of you here. The nurse will take you girls to the lab."

As they were leaving, Hannah teased Caitlin about having to have her blood drawn the old-fashioned way while Hannah could have hers taken from her central line.

Dr. Thornby explained why they wanted to be absolutely certain there really was a good match.

"The type of transplant depends on the source of the cells. If a patient donates his or her own cells, it's called autologous transplantation. If a patient had an identical twin, it would be a syngeneic transplantation. Since Hannah doesn't have an identical twin and wasn't able to donate her own cells, her only option is an allogeneic transplant from a sibling, a relative, or an unrelated donor. The reason it matters so much is related to the number of potential side effects, depending on who the donor is."

"I'm sure you know we already had the testing done at Maine Med," I said.

"Yes, I do, but we are being extremely careful and just want to verify that the antigen match is really as good as that test showed. If it is, then Hannah's body will be more likely to accept Caitlin's cells without rejection or a high risk of GVHD."

"You're talking about graft versus host disease, right?" I asked.

"That's correct. If GVHD occurred, Caitlin's cells would identify Hannah's cells as foreign and attack them, specifically skin, eyes, stomach, and intestines most commonly. The severity can range from mild to severe."

The test they planned to repeat now would be looking at the proteins on the surface of both Caitlin and Hannah's cells. The HLA (human leukocyte-associated antigens) test would look at how closely these antigens matched. Since there is usually only a 25 to 35% possibility of a sibling match, they wanted to retest to make certain the previous test wasn't in error. We talked briefly about the value of such a match and our own surprise that it had happened. We also talked about what Caitlin's role would be if they matched.

Dr. Thornby and Mike discussed the research Mike had found on the Internet along with statistical probabilities. Since I already knew in general about most of this on a theoretical level, I was content to just listen and take in all of the various research data that was being discussed. I reverted to the same attitude I had had about chemotherapy and treatment initially. My bottom line was how difficult it would be with the side effects on a day-to-day basis, and whether this procedure would significantly and decidedly raise her odds for long-term survival.

A couple of hours into the consultation, we came to a decision point, and Mike asked Dr. Thornby what for him was *the* crucial question: "Knowing all that you know in this field and understanding all of the research and statistical odds, if this were your child, what would you choose?"

Dr. Thornby said, "Given that she has done so well with chemotherapy, and the fact that she would definitely be sterile if she has to go through radiation therapy, I would probably choose to stay with the chemotherapy protocol and have the transplant as backup if she relapses."

With a stunned look on his face, Mike said, "Sterile?"

"I thought you knew that the radiation would definitely make her sterile, but she has at least a possibility of maintaining reproductive function with the chemotherapy, especially since she has been on the meds to suppress ovulation and control any possible bleeding problems," Dr. Thornby said.

Mike's eyes filled as he said, "I didn't really understand that. It changes the equation, especially since the odds of survival aren't that much different. If she does well with treatment, she has about a 68% chance of survival with chemotherapy and a 72% chance with radiation. It doesn't seem worth the small statistical advantage, does it?"

Dr. Thornby said, "Transplantation is statistically more effective with a higher certainty of survival, but there are tradeoffs in the higher incidence of complications from infection and the side effects from radiation."

"I'm mostly worried about the actual transplantation process, plus Hannah's been doing very well with the chemotherapy. The decision, if left totally up to me, would be to continue with chemotherapy," I said.

"Before, I would have said we should definitely do the transplant because the odds for cure were better, but now, I don't like the tradeoffs," Mike added.

Dr. Thornby said, "I can support what you're thinking and I'll contact Dr. Hurwitz to let him know you'll be returning to MMC. I'll send a report to them. I wish you well and hope she stays in remission."

As quickly as that, with the consult over, our decision had been made. We were going back MMC, which suddenly felt like going home. It was strange to think I was looking forward to being someplace I often dreaded returning to, but the alternative was definitely more frightening. I knew I would become accustomed to treatment here if it was necessary, but what had been alien at MMC prior to diagnosis was now a familiar landscape.

We went in search of Hannah and Caitlin and discovered that they had been given a tour of the clinic including the location of the cafeteria. It was lunchtime, and with a decision in hand, I was suddenly very hungry. As we ate lunch, the girls told of their adventures and we discussed what we learned from Dr. Thornby. Hannah said the decision was fine with her. I wasn't certain she completely understood the enormity of the choice, but she had faith and felt comfortable at MMC.

We were finally headed north to New Hampshire after struggling through midafternoon Boston traffic. I felt relieved to be out of the city, and during the hour's drive home, I closed my eyes and allowed our decision to percolate through my mind. I processed it through various internal centers, including my medical knowledge, my mom filter, and my gut-feelings center. All of them felt congruent. I relaxed and took a deep breath for the first time all day. For now, we were doing the best we could for Hannah. I didn't look forward to another round of chemotherapy, but at least I was clearer about our options.

"How do you feel now that we've made the decision?" I asked Mike.

"I think this is the right thing to do for now and I like that we have an option in our back pocket, so to speak. Dr. Thornby seemed very knowledgeable and honest about our options. I didn't feel as if he was selling any particular approach; he just had a lot of data. I think we covered all of the risks and the choices without pressure. It seems important not to choose something with more side effects and possible risks if we aren't forced to," he said.

"Yep. I'm glad that we both heard all of the data together. It would have been harder for me to try to explain it to you without the benefit of Dr. Thornby's knowledge of studies and results from places in England and Europe."

We both felt as if this was a well-thought-out decision. It felt good to be in agreement, and for the time being, our path was unambiguous. MMC would notify use about the third round of chemotherapy when it was time. We would take our chances with the side effects from chemotherapy, understanding she might still relapse. Wanting to enjoy the rest of the day, I put those thoughts aside and basked in the sounds of Hannah and Caitlin laughing and talking in the back seat. At the moment my life was good.

Ignoring the coming reality of returning to the hospital, we spent the rest of the week at the local outdoor pool. Hannah's counts were high enough to fight infection, and although she couldn't be in the pool because of her central line, she had a wonderful time hanging out reading and talking with her best friend Ellen Claire. We also played mini golf several times, laughing our way through every round. This was the kind of therapy all of us needed.

On Monday, August 26th, Hannah's ANC was high enough to start the third round of chemotherapy. The next day she would be readmitted; our idyll was over. The front hall was empty. Everything we needed for hospitalization was in the car except my emotional readiness.

While Hannah was going through the admission process, I hauled our bags in from the car. On my last trip to her room, I saw Dr. Hurwitz at the nurse's station.

"You must be really confused. The medical oncologists send you off to Boston for transplantation, and the surgical oncologists send you back here for the next round of chemotherapy and medical treatment," he said.

I laughed and said, "Dr. Thornby was great. We felt really good about all of the data and the decision-making process we went through with him. Not that we want to keep doing this, but we feel good about the decision."

"Good, we'll start the chemotherapy this evening," he said.

Premedication for nausea made Hannah drowsy. I sat holding her hand as she relaxed and slowly fell asleep. In keeping with my new plan to use all reasonable modalities to improve her chances of recovery and to try to prevent complications, I placed Dr. Andrew Weil's "Healing Sounds" CD into her CD player and placed the earphones over her ears. She wasn't convinced that it would help, but if it did, it would do the job while she was in dream sleep. I focused positive energy through Therapeutic Touch and quietly aligned her body with CST techniques as the chemotherapy slowly infused. After the infusion was completed, I focused healing thoughts and prayer on her body, visualizing her as a healthy vibrant eleven-year-old.

I believed these modalities had the potential to improve patient outcomes. A steadily growing number of recovery rooms and intensive care units were using Reiki healing therapy and Therapeutic Touch to speed recovery time and improve healing. If her chances of recovery were improved by these approaches, I was giving her a better chance.

With no complications during the night, they started the second dose of ARA-C the next morning. I was repeating my complementary therapies when Dr. Hurwitz came in to make rounds and check on her. He asked what it was I was doing and I explained my belief in these complementary therapies. He was curious, but supportive, asking if it worked for other things. I told him of my experiences and some of the results that I had heard about for other problems.

He told me he had broken his pinky toe over the weekend running barefoot. He was limping and it was painful, and he asked if any of this would help. I told him I would be happy to do a CST three point healing technique on his toe. He finished examining Hannah as she slept and then sat down for his own treatment. After a few minutes he reported less pain and a warm, pleasant feeling in his toe. If it helped healing, that would be great.

The weekend was devoted to morning and night ARA-C treatments. All was proceeding according to plan until Sunday evening when Hannah spiked a temperature of 101.2F. Thinking back to the second round complications, I could feel my spirits sag. Were we in for another nightmare round? Until we received the blood culture results the next day, we were in suspended animation. Luck was with us; the results were negative and I stopped holding my breath. The third round was done; we could go home until her counts went down and she needed the G shots to bring her ANC back up.

Clinic visits to MCCP in Scarborough for transfusions and blood work would be all we needed to do. Hannah could live in her own room. I could sleep in my own bed. We would all be together. I felt like dancing.

Even though I feared jinxing our luck, I contacted the school to begin the process of integrating Hannah's educational needs into our plans. The school, of course, knew how we were doing and had begun the process of an IEP (plan for a student with disabilities and special needs) for the fall. Her return to school had not been part of my thoughts during the summer. If she survived, we would cope with future needs as they occurred. Now the time had come to make arrangements for her to be coded with a disability. She couldn't attend school here, but while we were in the hospital, she could attend classes in the unit classroom with the teacher there. The school would decide if a tutor was needed. They would arrange for the middle school faculty to communicate with Hannah so she could complete assignments.

The Thursday after we came home from the hospital, one of the teachers from the sixth grade team Hannah was assigned to came with one of the guidance counselors to discuss what would be put in place. Hannah wouldn't be cleared to go to school until after she had completed chemotherapy and was again able to fight infections. We didn't know when that would be, but at least while she was at home now and when she was back in the hospital for the next round of chemotherapy, she would be included in the school process.

After they had talked with Hannah, the guidance counselor said that she had very good news. Caitlin's fifth grade teacher had retired, but was interested in doing some tutoring. She would be the liaison for us between Hannah's teaching team and the pediatric inpatient classroom teacher. Since we knew she was an excellent teacher, the whole process now seemed easier. She would pick up written assignments and leave them at our house for Hannah to complete. When Hannah was hospitalized, she would drop off assignments for the next week on Friday, so that I could take them with me on Monday. I would then return them so Hannah's work could be graded and credited. We would also have access to a laptop computer she could use in her room to e-mail assignments back to school. While I am certain she would have preferred being back with her class, this was a compromise that allowed her to keep up with sixth grade work during her treatment.

Caitlin was back in school, and I was thrilled to be here for her as she started her sophomore year. She would be playing on the varsity soccer team this fall, and I was avid to see as many games as I could. She was also still swimming with her club team, so she was very busy, but she couldn't wait to get home to see Hannah each day. The two of them sat together as Caitlin did her homework and Hannah read a book, if she had no school work.

My heart would fill and my eyes overflowed with tears every time I came upon them. I felt deep gratitude for two such wonderful people in my life. Although I didn't want what we were going through, I wondered if we would have developed these deep bonds without this experience. We would never know if our closeness as a family would have been so strong, but that strength and caring was what was allowing us to survive without being torn apart.

Chapter 19

BADLY SHAKEN

*Rigors: shaking chills in reaction to a severe infection or the release
of organisms, such as viruses or bacteria, into the bloodstream. An
abrupt attack of shivering and coldness, typically marking a rise in body
temperature at the onset of a fever.*

I was luxuriating in our time at home. Although I was surprised when
they told us we could be at home while her counts declined and then
built back up with the G shots, I wasn't looking a gift horse in the mouth.
Each day away from the hospital, at least pretending to lead normal lives,
was gratefully accepted. The quiet solitude of working in my garden
helped me to reconnect to home and the things I loved.

Even though Hannah relaxed and lazed through each day, a part
of her life was no different from being in the hospital. We started with
morning temperature checks, eye drops, and mouth care, and proceeded
to central line catheter flushes and dressing changes. A tray table beside
her bed sported sterile dressings, and underneath was the large box of
additional surgical supplies. For the daily flushes we assembled our pre-
filled syringes, masks, gloves, alcohol wipes, and the lock caps.

On the dressing change days, we had all of this plus our sterile field
tray, masks, gloves, dressing materials, and antiseptic cleaners. Hannah
was very comfortable with the whole procedure and became so adept at
flushing her ports that on most days I acted only in the role of supervising
nurse. She had discovered that if she wore a sports bra, she could keep
the two port catheters from dangling and pulling or getting caught on
anything. It also meant the dressing material had less tension on it and
tended not to need secondary tape to stay in place for the three days
between changes.

I tried to be as relaxed as Hannah was, but fear of a complication
tempered the elation I felt at being home. Attempting to fool the gods,
I superstitiously packed a bag with clean clothes; all we would need for

readmission was carefully arranged near the front door. Thankfully, so far, there was no evidence of any infection or skin breakdown. I fervently hoped we could stay home for the whole two or three weeks it took to recover her counts.

The days passed very quickly, and almost before I realized it, we had been home for a week. At our clinic visit, all of her blood work was what they expected as her counts dropped. She received platelets and saw the oncologist, who was encouraged by how she was doing. She looked good and was eating at home; having foods she loved had helped her not only feel better, but pack on an extra pound or two. I tended to cook according to what appealed to her, but also gave her a lot more variety than our sorties to local eating places in Portland allowed. She still loved my version of the Egg McMuffin, and some days would eat as many of four of these in addition to whatever else we were having. Her only regret was not being able to eat a BLT. Since she wasn't allowed any raw vegetables, she could only have the bacon part of the sandwich, which didn't appeal to her as much. At least she was able to have fresh-cooked vegetables from our garden, which made me feel better about what she was receiving nutritionally.

I had begun to let my guard down and worry less, but true to form in our experiences with cancer treatment, just when we thought the process was going smoothly, another complication occurred. I was used to Hannah awakening early, doing her care routine, and then wanting something to do. When she awoke late, ate only one egg muffin, and spent most of the morning sitting upstairs wrapped Indian style in her fuzzy blanket reading, listening to music, and resting, my radar went on high alert. Even though her temperature was normal when we checked it first thing in the morning, she seemed less energetic. I started checking her temperature every hour, but throughout the morning it remained a normal 98.6 degrees.

At noon, however, she only wanted some soup, so I re-checked her temperature and found it was up to 98.9 degrees. Although this wouldn't be much of a change in a healthy child, for one with a compromised immune system, I knew it might be the first signal that an infection was in the offing. After lunch, looking pale and exhausted, she went to bed and took a nap. Her temperature was now 99.0 degrees.

I called the pediatric inpatient unit and talked with one of the nurses. She said she would alert the oncologist at MCCP. She reminded me that if Hannah's temperature rose to 100.0 degrees, we needed to come to the hospital as quickly as possible. I started praying it wouldn't be an infection, but I needed to get everything ready just in case.

My eyes blurred with tears as I watched Hannah sleep with no hat covering her bald head. Her face was flushed and dark circles had formed under her eyes. I didn't think I was going to get my wish about staying home. I decided to let her sleep while I packed the car. At three o'clock, her temperature was 99.4 degrees. I updated MMC again and called Mike to tell him we were probably going to have to go back. Caitlin would stay here, and I called the people who gave her rides to swimming and her other activities. With the car packed, I awakened Hannah at 4:30. Her temperature was 100.2. I had to half carry her to the car. My heart pounded as I hoped I hadn't waited too long to leave. Caitlin hugged her and said, "I love you," as she helped put the seat back so that Hannah could lie down.

I called the ER to tell them we were on our way. They reminded me that if she started to go bad on the way, to head to the nearest ER to get an IV started on her central line. The nurse said they would expect us in about an hour and fifteen minutes. Alone in the car I listened to Hannah's breathing which was getting louder.

"Mom, I feel really bad," she whispered in a small, shaky voice.

"I know and I'm so sorry, sweetie. I'll get you there as fast as I can. As soon as they start the IV antibiotics, you'll start to feel better."

I wished I were as confident as I tried to sound.

All I could think about now was getting there, fast. Frustrated with the necessary slow speeds on the two-lane roads before reaching Interstate 95, I basically floored it once I was on the highway. I had never in my life driven 90 miles an hour, but I decided that if a cop stopped me, he could just escort me the rest of the way to the ER at MMC. Hannah was now very pale and her breathing was rapid. She felt hotter to the touch. My fear and the speed at which I was driving heightened my senses. I was attuned to every movement and sound she made. It was a race against infection and fever, and I intended to win. We just had to arrive at the ER before she got any worse.

I wheeled onto the parking apron in front of the ER entrance, my stomach twisting in knots. I tried not to let Hannah feel my nervousness as I kept talking calmly to her, telling her to hang in there, we would soon have her in bed. The parking valet took one look at her and agreed to take care of the car. I handed him the keys and got Hannah out of the car half carrying her through the ER doors. I grabbed the first wheelchair I saw and helped her sit down. My heart sank when I saw how crowded the waiting area was. Putting aside decorum and politeness, I pushed ahead of people at the check-in; today I didn't care. I wanted her upstairs as quickly as possible.

When I gave the triage nurse Hannah's name, she said, "Wow, we didn't expect you for another twenty minutes. You must have flown."

I nodded, unable to make small talk. She handed me over to the clerk who would take our insurance information. I stood tapping my foot as she fiddled with various papers, seemingly uninterested in our interaction.

"I don't mean to be rude, but my daughter needs to be admitted to the pediatric unit to have an IV antibiotic started as quickly as possible."

She looked up, stared at me as if I had spoken in a foreign language, and went back to finding a clipboard. I shifted from foot to foot wanting to pace. I knelt down by Hannah, felt her forehead, and took her pulse, which was very rapid. Finally the woman made a copy of our insurance card and went off to create a wrist band. As soon as she was done, I grabbed the ID band from her hand and didn't wait for a transporter as I pushed Hannah's wheelchair toward the elevators at a run.

On the pediatric unit, they were waiting for us. One of the nurses assisted Hannah into bed, where she curled up into a ball. Blood cultures were drawn from her central line and an IV antibiotic was hung according to protocol. They hooked Hannah up to a continuous vital signs monitor in case her blood pressure went too low or her fever went too high. I answered all the admission questions as I rubbed Hannah's back and reassured her that she would feel better soon. I kept checking the vital signs monitor and saw her temperature had jumped to 103.

Hannah grabbed my arm and said, "Mom I feel really bad. My head hurts. I'm gonna be sick!"

Eyes wide with fear, her body contorted as she shook and shivered. The bed rattled. Her teeth chattered. The monitor read 104.5 degrees. The nurse grabbed all the blankets she had and covered her. I jerked down the side rail and crawled into her bed, adding my warmth. Her tears wet my shirt as rigors wracked her body. Two or three long minutes later, the spasms subsided.

Mumbling through still partially clenched teeth, she said, "Mom, my legs hurt so much, I feel like I've been running for a long time."

She tried to open her jaw, but the pain started a fresh flood of tears.

I held her.

"Try to take some slow deep breaths to help relax your muscles. That was pretty awful, wasn't it, buggy?"

"I don't ever want to do that again," she said.

"You and me both, kiddo! The antibiotics and pain medication should start working and then you'll feel better. Just rest and try to sleep for now."

She nodded as her eyes closed and her face and body gradually relaxed into sleep. Once I was certain she was asleep and, for the moment, stable, I got up. I hated to leave her for even one minute, but I needed to get the car and bring in our belongings. It looked as if we were back in the hospital for a while.

Her nurse patted my shoulder and said, "Knowing about rigors and seeing it are two different things, aren't they?"

"Yeah, it's so counter-intuitive when someone is burning up with fever that you put covers on them, but I guess shaking chills is the right name," I said.

"It's the abrupt temperature spike that seems to cause it. Yeah, it does seem the wrong thing to do, but it works to stabilize them," she said.

As I walked to the elevator, I thought about what a close call this had been. I had now learned firsthand about rigors. Simply knowing that someone with a compromised immune system who couldn't fight infection was susceptible was different from experiencing it. Another enemy was on my radar.

The after-effects of adrenaline were making me shaky. I knew I would need to sit down soon so my legs wouldn't give way beneath me, but first I needed to move the car to long-term parking. Feeling like a pack mule, I hauled everything upstairs and collapsed onto the parent bed. My world had once again become the size of a hospital room with only one focus…Hannah.

Despite the terrible experience of the rigors, the next day Hannah had no fever, and although she was sore from the muscles spasms, she didn't feel ill. They couldn't explain the cause; the blood cultures were negative and she didn't spike any more fevers. We resumed our old patterns for living in the hospital with my only regret being not having my bicycle. Instead I drove to the Back Bay estuary area at 5 A.M. and ran three miles. I didn't enjoy running, but it kept me sane and gave me a good workout.

Five days later, despite Hannah's counts being at their lowest, they let us go home again and start the G shots. The normal precautions of hand-washing, isolation from anyone who was sick, and careful monitoring of her temperature would be enough until she could fight infections again.

Once home, I greedily took advantage of every opportunity I had to attend Caitlin's soccer games and any of her other school activities. It was a relief to be a mom in only one place. What had seemed hectic with swim practice every day and varsity soccer practice and games now felt infinitely doable, as long as I could be here at home. I knew it would be a short-lived reprieve, but I wasn't going to complain as long as Hannah didn't develop another fever or have any other problems.

We no longer had the cleaning service, but being able to be home for more than a weekend allowed me to keep up with the house. I cooked future meals for Mike and Caitlin and put them in the freezer. In fact, being in control of my own household again was very therapeutic. Doing mindless tasks that were also productive was definitely more relaxing than the constant strain of living in the hospital.

Worry still rode my shoulders like a familiar yoke, but in many respects I had learned to stop thinking about what could go wrong next. It was a very subtle shift in my world view. Initially, I had felt powerless before Hannah was hospitalized and during the first part of treatment. While I was still powerless in many ways, I felt less so. I had regained my ability to advocate for her, use my nursing and medical knowledge, and now had confidence in our ability to survive whatever was going to be thrown at us next. I wasn't being fatalistic; it was more that I now accepted that we would continue to face challenges until her treatments were done. Worrying about them when they weren't happening was exhausting and only served to reduce my ability to cope.

Hannah lived in the moment. If she felt well, she was up and doing whatever entertained her. If she felt bad, she went to bed and accepted whatever had to be done to make her feel better. I continued to learn important life lessons from this amazing eleven-year-old.

Chapter 20
UNABLE TO RESIST

Imunno-compromised: lacking a fully effective immune system. Most frequently seen in patients receiving chemotherapy, which makes them susceptible to organisms which would not cause illness in the normal, healthy individual.

To my surprise, while we were home after the third round of chemotherapy, Hannah's hair grew back---but it wasn't blond, straight, and fine; it was coarse, black and curly. She found her new hair funny, but had mixed feelings about not having long blond hair anymore. For now she was just happy that it was growing back in so soon.

No one could fully explain why, when you lost your hair to chemotherapy, it grew back a different color and texture. One of the nurses told us of one family who all had very black curly hair, but when their child's hair grew back in it was platinum blond and completely straight. For most people, the hair returns to its normal color and texture in a year, but not always.

I wondered if a permanent change in hair color could alter who we were. Certainly people dyed their hair and felt differently about themselves. Would Hannah relate to the world in a different way if she had black hair? Would the world relate differently to Hannah if she had black hair? In Hannah's mind this may have been more important than it was to me right now. I didn't know how I would feel if the hair change was permanent, but it was one of those things I refused to worry about. First she needed to survive; then we would worry about the details.

Unless Hannah developed a fever or some other complication, we would only be at MMC for two or three days to have the first part of the fourth round of chemotherapy. She would once again have the ARA-C, but since they had not been able to give the Danorubicin in the second round as planned, it would be given now. What had seemed intimidating and strange when we first started, now was commonplace. It was hard to believe that we had been doing this since the end of May, eighteen weeks ago.

We moved back into the small positive-pressure room. I didn't anticipate any problems with this round, so hadn't brought most of our stuff with us. Hannah was feeling good going into this hospitalization with close to normal blood counts. I thought again about what Dr. Thornby had said about how she looked compared to what her medical record showed, and allowed myself a sliver of hope.

We had come in on Wednesday and if all went well, we could leave on Friday, September 27th. I looked forward to being home again so quickly. After the last dose of chemotherapy finished on Thursday evening, Hannah was sleepy from medication and didn't want to eat much. I didn't think much of it until during the night the nausea continued long after the chemo was done. Even with continued doses of antinausea medication, she felt sick. The fact that we had avoided a problem like this until this fourth round had pushed the possibility from my mind. I guess we had just been lucky up to this point.

As I packed up our personal items for home, I talked with Gail, Hannah's nurse, about the choices we had for dealing with this. After discussion with the on-call oncologist, arrangements were made for a prescription for the antinausea medication to give around the clock at home. She could also take the Benadryl, which had the dual benefits of decreasing nausea and making her sleep.

I loaded the car with what little we had brought with us while they completed discharge paperwork. Hoping to prevent vomiting on the ride home, I asked Gail to medicate her just before we left the unit. She agreed, and had just finished administering the medication intravenously when I came back from bringing the car to the front of the hospital. As soon as the central lines were flushed, we got ready to leave, but for the first time in all of our discharges, Hannah needed a wheelchair. As I pushed the wheelchair to the car, my only thought was to arrive home as soon as possible.

Curled around the pink wash basin at her side, she lay down and closed her eyes. I patted her back as I tuned the radio to MPBN and was happy to hear a piano concerto by Beethoven. I hoped the classical music would be soothing enough for her to at least rest, if not sleep.

We usually broke up the drive home with a stop at the Kennebunk rest area, which had bathroom facilities. When we got there, I got out, but Hannah insisted she didn't need to use the bathroom. I raced inside and was thankful there was no line for a toilet. As I rushed back to the parking lot, I saw an elderly couple staring at our car. I ran forward until I could see what they were staring at. Hannah was vomiting into her pink basin, looking very miserable.

I opened the door and held the basin.

"Do you want to go inside to rinse out your mouth and clean up a bit?"

"No. Please just empty my bucket and bring me some water."

"Are you sure you don't need the bucket again right away?"

"I'm okay now."

She sighed and lay back down in the seat.

I handed her a water bottle so she could rinse her mouth and a wet-wipe to clean up a bit. Everything had gone into the basin, so that was a blessing. I hurried inside with the basin half full of the lunch she had eaten a couple of hours ago. After cleaning the basin, I bought her another bottle of water and ran back to the car. She wasn't due for any more medication yet, so I hoped she might be able to sleep and we could make it home without more vomiting.

As we turned into the driveway at home thirty minutes later, Hannah sat up, grabbed the pink basin, and vomited again. I helped her into the house when she was finished, and after she had washed up and cleaned out her mouth, I tucked her into her own bed after a dose of Benadryl.

Laughing, she said, "Well, that is one thing I probably won't want to eat anytime soon. Once you have seen macaroni and cheese in one of those pink buckets, it definitely loses its appeal."

"I can certainly understand that!" I couldn't believe her sense of humor after what she had just been through.

"Mom did you know that I made up my mind when we left the hospital I wouldn't throw up until we were at least halfway home?"

"Really?"

"Yep, I thought if I could make it halfway before I threw up, I would be okay. I made it to Kennebunk first and then I decided I'd try to make it home before I had to puke again. And I did!"

I pulled her into my arms.

"You're such a strong kid. It takes a lot of mental toughness to be able to do that. There aren't a lot of adults who would be able to do it. You're so great!"

She snuggled down under the covers to sleep. I took a quick drive to the pharmacy to pick up her prescription, unloaded the car when I got back, and started the laundry. Even though this wouldn't be a long visit home, I hoped the nausea would get better and we could stay the full four days without any complications or a fever.

Summer had come and gone. As I lay in bed that night, I thought back over the past weeks, our missed summer. My garden, which had always been a place of solace and meditation, was ready for winter thanks to the help of friends. I had planted the garden before Hannah was diagnosed, but then had only been able to spend a few precious, therapeutic days on my hands and knees weeding. Spending most of my time in a hospital room had robbed me of a feeling of connection with nature and the seasons. My walks and bike rides had helped, but now, with less daylight, that would be harder. I needed to find a way to maintain my well-being once we returned to the hospital for what I hoped would be the last chemo treatment.

Knowing we would be in the hospital again for a longer period of time, I brought all of our room decorations. While Dr. Hamilton admitted Hannah, I fixed up the room. When I was finished, everything in the room looked cheerful except for its occupant; she was curled up in a ball on her bed looking miserable.

We hadn't solved the nausea problem. This was going to be a very unpleasant couple of weeks if they couldn't fix it, but there was hope. Dr. Hamilton explained they had a new drug that could work. The only problem was the cost, and the need for prior insurance approval. They wanted to hold off on starting the chemotherapy until they tried this drug. Thankfully, within a day or two they succeeded in obtaining the preauthorization, and the drug did significantly decrease the nausea.

There was more good news. Once the two days of ARA-C were completed, WE WERE DONE WITH CHEMO! The initial road map had planned for five rounds, but we were done after only four. Did that mean that Hannah had done better than they expected? Perhaps we were lucky after all!

I called Mike.

"Guess what?"

"Nothing bad happened, did it?"

"Nope. Good news. We are done with chemo after the next two days of ARA-C!"

"Seriously?"

"Yep. I could dance, but I'm afraid to jinx us."

"Yeah, let's wait until we're home and she's fine to celebrate, but I'm happy she did better than originally planned. Give Hannah a big hug and tell her good job."

"Will do. Talk to you later."

I really was excited, but knew we had to get through this without complications. We fell back into our old hospital routines with the only difference being I was running around the Back Bay marginal way instead of riding my bike. I was more relaxed than I had been for any previous round of therapy, feeling more than ready to cope with what appeared to be a very straightforward hospitalization. Hannah had become so used to the routine that once the nausea problem was improved, she went to the unit classroom, did school assignments and hung out in the playroom if she felt well.

Several artists came to the unit to paint pictures on the glass windows into the hallways to brighten up each room. These were mostly pictures of favorite characters from movies or TV. Hannah instead requested a picture of Larry, her neon-green-and-purple alligator, which made her room uniquely hers. She had her favorite quilts and blankets on her bed exactly the way she wanted them, creating a home space that was hers alone. Now her marine-themed room was complete; it would have been a great place to hang out except for the IV pump and other hospital equipment.

In the larger positive-pressure room next to us was the little girl who also had AML. She had suffered no permanent damage from the life-threatening infection and other than needing to keep the shunt patent that protected her brain from fluid buildup, was doing great. The treatment schedule had been delayed, so this was her fourth and last round as well. Her mother asked me what we were doing for Hannah's celebration for the last day of chemotherapy. It wasn't a tradition I was familiar with, but I was informed that the child picked the menu and shared with the doctors and nurses.

I discussed it with Hannah, who announced she wanted my homemade tuna casserole as her celebration food. She couldn't tolerate sweets and wanted no cake or ice cream. I thought, *At least she has her own unique ideas.* She wanted to share it with the staff and any of the other families who were there, though I was pretty certain they wouldn't be as thrilled with this choice as Hannah was. Now all I had to do was figure out a way to provide this repast.

I asked Liz if the Ronald McDonald House would let me cook there. She contacted them and they were happy to oblige. I walked to the grocery store, where I did my usual shopping while we were in Portland, and got all of the ingredients. Now we just needed for Hannah to tolerate these last two days of chemotherapy without complications.

I spent the morning as Hannah was receiving her last dose of chemotherapy making the casserole. I made two pans of it, not knowing who would want some and who wouldn't. It smelled delicious to me, and although the staff at the Ronald McDonald House was bemused by Hannah's choice, they said that they felt Hannah was lucky to have a mom who could cook for her. I thanked them and felt guilty that I wasn't making this for the people staying there as well. When I arrived on the pediatric unit laden with the two pans of tuna casserole wrapped in towels to keep them warm, Hannah was feeling awake enough to be hungry for lunch. We invited the staff and any patient families who wanted to participate into her room to share in her celebration.

Several people tried the tuna casserole, but it certainly wasn't cake and ice cream. Those who had the courage to try some declared it very good, which pleased Hannah. As for me, I didn't really care about anyone but Hannah. She loved it and that was celebration enough for me. Our little party was short and evoked mixed feelings. We had struggled so hard to reach this point, now that we had arrived, I was at a loss about what happened next. I had to fight back tears as the staff gave her little gifts and remembrances for the end of chemo. There was too, too much of the casserole, so I wrapped it up in meal-size portions and put it in the freezer in the family-room kitchen. She could have what was left anytime she felt like it.

As I prepared to leave for the weekend, I felt hopeful about our chances of making it through this without severe complications and long-term disabilities. I kissed her goodbye and saw her anew. She looked like the kids in the Journey of Hope book I hadn't wanted to read so many months ago. Her round, puffy face, eyes made prominent by deep circles, a thin body and at times a bald head gave her that same cancer-patient appearance. I peered into her eyes and saw an ancient soul who had lost all semblance of childhood innocence. It hadn't just been five months for her, but a lifetime.

She had completely missed her eleven-year-old summer. Her life was bordered by where she was in treatment, how much stamina she had, and whether her blood counts were high enough to fight infection. She had started this as a child, but she would never be able to return to being a child again. My heart ached for her lost innocence and shortened childhood. While I mourned the loss, I knew that if she survived, I would gladly trade her innocence and childhood for recovery. As long as she was here with us, I didn't care if she looked like a cancer patient.

By this time, the nursing staff was used to the differences between Mike and me when we lived in Hannah's room. The weekends were relaxed and full of anything fun they could think to do. Mike even brought in a soccer ball and was teaching some of the kids to dribble in the halls. One weekend when Dr. Schwenn was on call, her husband brought their five-year-old daughter in so that they could all eat dinner together, and Mike proceeded to introduce the girl to soccer by having her learn to dribble around Hannah's IV pole. He had Hannah making long circuits around the unit pushing her IV pole for some exercise whenever she felt well enough, and they watched lots of movies. He reread the *Lord of the Rings* trilogy to her and started another fantasy series.

Even though I wanted her room clean and organized and daily routines maintained, I too loved watching an occasional movie with her. Our favorite was *The Fellowship of the Ring*. One evening as we watched it, I listened with a new sensitivity to a poignant exchange between Frodo and Gandalf.

As Frodo struggles with his burden of trying to return the ring to Mount Doom to be destroyed, he says, "I wish the ring had never come to me. I wish none of this had happened."

Gandalf replies, "So do all who live to see such times. All we have to decide is what to do with the time that is given to us."

This quote seemed to sum up exactly what we were experiencing. We hadn't been given a choice and we heartily wished it had never happened. The only choice we had was to decide what to do with the time given us. I thought long and hard that night about all of the energy I was spending on what-ifs. Although this was hard, we were choosing how to spend the time we were given, and in this experience it was on a day-by-day, sometimes hour-by-hour basis. I needed to take every opportunity to love and appreciate Hannah and my family, not for what they could give me, but for the very fact that I was fortunate enough to have them in my life, no matter how much time we had together.

Hannah's counts dropped rapidly, and to her dismay, so did her new hair. The worst part was that it fell out in oddly spaced clumps around her head. The nurses told her it was the result of having the Danorubicin again, but whatever the cause, she was back to wearing hats even when she was asleep.

With her platelets depleted from the chemo, she began receiving transfusions again. Since she was always medicated for this, she slept. One afternoon after a transfusion, she awoke around 4 P.M. not feeling good. Her nurse took her temperature; it was 99.4F. She notified the oncologist and began frequent vital signs checks. In less than an hour, Hannah had a fever of 101.5F. Blood cultures were drawn and an IV antibiotic was started.

A few minutes later Hannah said, "Mom, I'm going to be sick."

I grabbed her basin and helped her lean over the side of the bed as she vomited. I rang for her nurse, who came in to empty the basin. As I turned to take the basin back, Hannah grabbed my arm and started to cry as she began to shake. The nurse ran to get more blankets and I crawled into bed with Hannah and held her as she went into another episode of rigors. I added my warmth to the blankets that swaddled her and held her until the spasms stopped. *This stinks*, I thought, and would have liked to have joined my tears to hers.

She was started on acetaminophen for pain relief, sleep, and fever control. She had no fever the next time they checked her, and after 9 P.M. she felt fine and was able to sleep comfortably. I didn't sleep. My thoughts were focused on blood culture results with the hope that they wouldn't find anything, but somewhere in my deepest, darkest thoughts, I knew this might be bad news. All of my self-assurance about sailing through this last hospitalization was in jeopardy.

Hannah awoke the next day feeling fine and the blood cultures came back negative. We still needed to wait for the 48 and 72 hour results, but my hopes soared as I heard the news on rounds. Perhaps I was being too pessimistic. Hannah certainly didn't seem ill; her appetite was fine, and other than being tired from her low blood counts, she was able to do school work and, with a mask on, attend class.

I crashed back to an unpleasant reality, my optimism short-lived, when the 72 hour culture results showed gram positive rods. There were so few colonies, they needed to allow them to grow longer. The final results wouldn't be available until the next week. I maintained a faint hope it would turn out to be some contaminate. I didn't talk with Hannah much about it as I didn't want to either discourage her or raise her hopes. Instead I focused on foraging for whatever she wanted to eat, which at the moment was enormous quantities of scoop corn chips with Newman's Own Salsa.

When the cultures had finally grown, the news wasn't good. They were still trying to confirm the exact organism, but it seemed to be very rare. For now they were leaning toward nocardia, an inhaled organism that causes lesions in the lungs. The resulting pulmonary abscesses could then easily spread throughout the body, especially to the liver, brain, and kidneys. Nocardia was hard to kill and had a tendency to be in remission for a while and then became worse again. Most people would not be at risk---only those with compromised immune systems, such as HIV patients and children receiving chemotherapy.

A whole new cast of characters began showing up on medical rounds: the Infectious Disease specialists (ID). They came to examine Hannah and quiz us about any exposure to dirt. Since we had been in the positive-pressure room, I had no idea how Hannah had come in contact with an inhaled organism from dirt, but if it was this organism, the real question was would they be able to treat it, and how would treatment affect our being in the hospital. My visions of what might occur from here on were nightmarish.

Once again she would lose her central line. I understood why they were being so cautious, but it was very discouraging. Without her central line, all of our problems with peripheral IVs were back. Hannah was discouraged and depressed. She didn't want to go to surgery again and she especially didn't like the thought of how inconvenient and painful things would be without her central line. We were losing something that made Hannah's treatment tolerable for her.

As we waited for surgery on Friday morning, my mood was black. All hopes of getting out of this last round of therapy easily had vanished. The ID specialists, as well as CDC were still researching which exact organism it might be. Hannah was on antibiotics that needed CDC approval before they could be given. Looking at her, I couldn't see any evidence of her being ill, and I still couldn't imagine how it was that she had been exposed to this in the hospital in an isolation room.

By the middle of the next week, the ID doctors had agreed on a final diagnosis. They had a great deal of difficulty with growing the organism in the lab, but they believed that her central line was infected with an organism called Tsukamurella *tyrosinosolvens*, which had been isolated by a Japanese researcher in the ovaries of ladybugs. I sat staring at them in disbelief as they told me what they had decided. How in the world had a ladybug's ovaries with some strange organism in them gotten inside Hannah's central line? It seemed totally preposterous. With the exception of one article in the medical literature, there was no information on it. The organism was in the same family as nocardia and had been isolated from the sputum of patients with chronic pulmonary disease, who were imunno-compromised. There had only been one child diagnosed with the *tyrosinosolvens* type of the Tsukamurella species and that child also had AML.

We began to see researchers and post-doctoral fellows in their stiff white lab coats on rounds with the ID doctors. I thought, cynically, *Well, at least you will all be able to be part of a published paper on this rare situation because you examined Hannah.*

As one of them interviewed us, my anger at all that was happening converted to some nasty sarcasm, and I said, "Gee, Hannah. I guess you'll have to stop eating so many lady bugs as snacks."

He spun around to look at me and said, "Does she really eat ladybugs as snacks?"

I spat back, "Of course she doesn't."

His face fell and he said, "Oh, you were joking."

At that point, I knew I was close to losing my temper and being extremely rude. This was potentially a disastrous complication for my daughter. After surviving the chemotherapy, she might now have some untreatable infectious disease that could eventually kill her. My rage boiled up from deep inside and I wanted to throw things at people and have a tantrum. I wanted to scream at these people, blame someone or, better yet, hit someone, but I didn't. I excused myself and went to the bathroom, sat in the dark crying, trying to breathe, and hoping for some reprieve from this newest ogre we had to fight.

They never found the source of the infection or how it got into her central line; all of the cultures from the central line linings, tips, and cuff were negative. There was no evidence that it was really infected. A medical student offered what I thought was perhaps the most plausible explanation of all. There could have been a ladybug in the lab that walked across the agar plate and laid an egg. I liked the humor behind the idea, even if the science might not be accurate. From then on we referred to Hannah's infection as the ladybug ovary disease or as *suko tyrannosaurus.*

Even though we tried to joke about why she had to stay in the hospital, my sense of humor had fled. I was split again. With Hannah I tried to be cheerful and upbeat, but alone, I was down. I didn't want my mood to affect Hannah, worrying that if she became depressed, it could further weaken her already suppressed immune system. I had to find some humor or something to help us cope with this latest disaster. We were here until they decided she wasn't infected anymore, and no one would tell us how long that might be.

The days in the hospital moved so slowly it felt as if time ran backward. I still tried to get down to the Back Bay to walk or run, but it didn't help my mood at all. Hannah went to the unit classroom, did school work, and was bored and down.

Even with negative results from the central line and peripheral veins, the plan didn't change. The ongoing negative cultures verified my skepticism about whether she really had an infection, as they claimed. After a couple of days of feeling victimized by the situation, I decided to ask if we could leave on a pass. Hannah's blood counts were returning to a level that allowed her fight any other infections, and she was on very strong antibiotics. I felt that time away would actually help her immune system, and she needed to see something other than the inside walls of a hospital.

All of our activity had to be bracketed by when the IV antibiotics were infused, so I worked out a schedule with the nursing staff to have her morning antibiotic finished by noon and the next one set for 4:30. This gave us several hours to be out. Initially, Hannah still tired very easily, so we just drove to some of the sightseeing places like the Portland Headlight, several smaller lighthouses, and the Old Port. As she regained strength, we ventured to places like the Portland Museum of Art where we enjoyed the current art show and had afternoon tea. We toured an historic sea captain's house and went to a local bookstore. We drove to Deering Oaks Park and walked to the small lake to see the duck house on an island in the middle. We even went to a matinee and saw the movie *VegiTales*. Unfortunately, to Hannah's embarrassment, I fell asleep during the movie and snored; not my most stimulating movie experience.

As we became more daring, we ventured farther away, going as far south as the estuary in Scarborough, where we had the good fortune to see a gray seal feeding in the one of the channels. It seemed a good omen to me, and I was cheered by the experience for several days afterward.

On one of our trips to the downtown bookstore, we parked across the street from a large church. As we got out of the car, Hannah asked, "Mom, are churches open so that you can go inside?"

"I don't know about this one, but some of them are. Do you want to find out if this one is?"

"Yeah, let's go see."

We crossed the street, entering the churchyard through the wrought-iron gates in the fence surrounding the beautiful old red brick buildings, and walked toward the lighted entrance. At the church office, we asked if the sanctuary was open. The secretary looked us over, then immediately said that she would be happy to show us the sanctuary and turn on more lights if we wanted them. Hannah said she didn't want any lights other than the ones on the altar. We sat down in a pew about halfway back and admired the vaulted ceiling and the stained-glass windows.

Hannah snuggled up close to me and asked, "Mom, can we have a little service for Andrea?"

For a moment I couldn't speak.

Finally I found my voice, "What a lovely idea, sweetie. I think that would be a very nice way to say goodbye to her."

I thought, *She barely knew that girl.* She had only spoken with her that one time when the girl was waiting for X-ray, and she had only played with the girl's sister in the playroom a few times. Hannah hadn't talked about her feelings at the time. Since it had happened back in July, I was surprised that it was still on her mind. The girl's death had obviously affected Hannah deeply, but she hadn't mentioned it.

We leafed through the prayer book, found a couple of passages that Hannah liked, and sang a couple of hymns. Between tears we talked.

"Do you think Andrea is an angel, Mom? I do."

"I wouldn't be at all surprised."

"I think God takes good people when they die and they become angels and helpers for God," she said.

"That's a good thing to believe, and it would make their families feel better since they are so sad from losing them."

"Yeah, I think so too," she said.

We sat with our arms around each other in comfortable silence, content with our own thoughts.

For the hundredth time since this had all started, I thought about how blessed I was to have this child whose immense beauty and wisdom enriched my life. I was grateful we had come in here, but sad that she knew so much about grief and loss so young. Slowly we walked, with our arms around each other, back to the churchyard. Our trip had started out as a mission to find a new book to read and ended up being a different journey of discovery. The books we picked out that day came to represent a very special experience. Each time I saw them, I was transported to that moment of intimacy, grateful for one more gift from this journey through Hannah's treatment.

Chapter 21
BEYOND THE RAINBOW

Transition: a process or period in which something
undergoes a change of status or condition.

As the days of late October shortened and became darker, so did my temper and mood. With each succeeding round of chemotherapy, it had taken longer for Hannah's bone marrow to return to normal. After the third round, it had only come back to a low normal level. This time it was even slower, but her ANC levels indicated we could be at home now were it not for the intravenous antibiotic therapy dominating our days.

I knew I should feel grateful that she was finished with chemotherapy and was still in remission, but instead I was frustrated and angry that we were still living at the hospital. The around-the-clock doses of super-antibiotics were causing problems with her veins. Every three days, hospital policy dictated changing the IV insertion site to protect her from developing phlebitis, which could cause infection. Her arms and hands were bruised and painful. Several of her veins were so inflamed that they needed continuous warm packs to decrease the redness and swelling. She was running out of veins for both the IV insertions and blood drawing. Both of us were losing patience.

To combat our frustration and depression, we continued to make forays into the outside world, and had gone as far a Caitlin's school in South Berwick, Maine, for a soccer game. I had asked the nurses if there was a limit to the distance we could go, or whether our outings were time-controlled only. They only cared about her being back for the late-afternoon dose of antibiotics, so we made the morning dose a little later and stayed long enough to watch Caitlin's game. Hannah sat bundled up in a blanket on the sidelines and read a book during part of the game, but she was happy to be where Caitlin was. Caitlin was thrilled that Hannah came, and my spirits soared. Oh, to only be doing such mundane things again.

We had also tried to work around the family separation by taking Caitlin to Portland on the weekends if we could manage it with school and sports schedules. On a beautiful Sunday at the end of October, I brought Caitlin with me so we could all go to Mackworth Island where the Baxter State School for the Deaf is located. A footpath encircling the island allows visitors a beautiful walk.

As we set out along the trail, I felt as if I had been invited to a feast for the senses. The foliage was at its peak, with rich crimsons and deep yellows on the maple and beech trees. A tangy scent of saltwater filled the air, and the warm sun glistened on the waters of the bay turbulent with schooling herring. Low-flying birds flocked over the shimmering waters, scooping up the tiny fish as they broke the surface in their frantic jostling. I had the video camera running as I followed Hannah and Caitlin walking with their arms around each other, deep in conversation. I was trying to capture these moments of joy. I wanted this to be our world---sunny, vibrant, teeming with life.

The walk was the longest Hannah had taken in months, but with Caitlin beside her, she made it all the way around the island. We sat in silence in the car, joined in gratitude for the gift of this day. We drove slowly back to the hospital, trying to make it last as long as we could.

Each day on rounds, I queried the ID doctors about being discharged and ending the high-powered antibiotics. Hannah had been through an episode of thrush (yeast infection) in her mouth already. I knew her body was being affected by the drugs, and I feared that they might do more harm than the chemotherapy had done. Were we fated to survive the cancer and succumb to complications from the treatment of a purported infection? I didn't want to burn any bridges or second-guess the experts, but I knew Hannah. I wondered if their knowledge was aimed more at research, than at caring for a real child. The last five weeks had been long and tedious. She needed to be out of a clinical environment.

Finally, they began to waver in their insistence that Hannah would need to stay in the hospital for an indefinite amount of time. The oncologists were ready for her to be released. Her ANC was at an acceptable level, and she was clearly showing signs of "hospitalitis." She was bored, and having to stay in this environment wasn't conducive to moving on after cancer treatment. There was no evidence of further infection and no real evidence that she had ever really had the dreaded "ladybug ovary disease." Perhaps I was being a wimp about all of this. Other families had spent years in the hospital with their children and they kept on going, but this felt as if there was no definitive reason for staying.

All weekend at home, I argued back and forth with myself. If she did have this infection, she had gotten it while in the hospital. Therefore, wouldn't home be a safer place? What if she really did have it and I wasn't able to recognize a worsening condition? But on the other hand, thinking logically, she would probably have fevers or a cough or skin changes, if she did begin to develop symptoms. If I knew what to look for, I was certain that I had the clinical skills to assess it. I could do IVs at home and whatever else it took.

By Monday morning my clinical side and mom side were in agreement. The oncologists were confident she was okay, but the infectious disease doctors were still concerned that she would somehow abruptly become very ill with this strange infection that had only been seen in one other person. Every fellow and resident in the Infectious Disease Department had examined her and agreed there was no evidence of systemic illness or lung or skin problems.

Seeing their hesitancy, I pounced, pitching my arguments about how detrimental it was for her to be here at risk, bored and quickly becoming more and more depressed about being in the hospital with no discharge date in sight. I reiterated my belief that depression could adversely affect her immune system while I assured them that I could infuse the IV antibiotics at home as long as we had the equipment. Critical Care Systems could provide the IV bags of antibiotics and the pump, and they would be able to do the blood draws and provide support for her care at home. It would certainly be cheaper than the cost of being here, even if they came every day.

Then I held my breath while they huddled, arguing back and forth. The decision: Hannah could go home with a peripheral IV! Inside I danced a jig; externally I behaved with professional decorum, looking serious and responsible. Critical Care Systems would provide the supplies for the IVs. She would be switched to oral Septra DS for the next six months, which would protect her against the possibility of pneumocystis carinii, a pneumonia which affects imunno-compromised patients. The Amicacin would continue to be via intravenous infusion to cover the possibility that she still had the Tsukamurella *tyrosinosolvens*.

Hannah jumped around in her bed in excitement, and began packing up all her bed friends and special blankets. I had everything ready to go in under twenty minutes. Snow was predicted for later in the day and I used that as an excuse to insist we leave by one o'clock. Part of me wanted to linger over goodbyes to everyone on the staff who had been so good to us, but I wanted to escape before they changed their minds. With cheers and waves, we loaded a wheelchair full of our belongings and headed for the door, hoping to only see everyone again when we came as visitors.

We had arrived in the beginning heat of summer; we were leaving in the beginning cold of winter. By the time we got to the York/Portsmouth, area the snow was heavy and I was glad we had left when we did. I breathed a sigh of relief as we stopped at the bottom of our unplowed driveway. Our snow-covered yard was a crystalline white wonderland. Initially, neither of us moved, savoring this moment of arriving home with no scheduled hospitalizations looming; then we just held hands and smiled.

I sat on the couch in front of the fireplace glowing with warmth and wallowing in the joy of being home. Hannah had reestablished permanence in her room, even though she had to share it with an IV pump. The refrigerator door was filled with the carefully labeled IV bags delivered by Critical Care Systems. Since the antibiotics needed to be infused every six hours, I arranged the administration times so that the doses would be on a 10 and 4 schedule. This would allow us the middle of the day free for activity and a five-hour block of sleep in the middle of the night. I didn't have any trouble waking up at 4 A.M., and since the IV pump beeped when it was finished, I could go back to bed for an hour while it was infusing and rise at my usual 5:00.

On the third day home, the IV site needed to be changed. After much back-and-forth phone discussion between us, ID, and MCCP, the IV antibiotics were replaced with oral treatment. Our final tie to the hospital routine was ended with less difficulty than I had anticipated. Almost as rapidly as she had started treatment, she had transitioned to post-treatment status. Hannah's sense of humor returned, and bubbles of laughter from somewhere deep inside me caused my feet to dance at unexpected moments.

Our social worker, Liz, and a couple of nurses from MCCP visited the middle school and met with all of the students who were in classes with Hannah. They presented information on AML and answered the time-honored question about whether anyone else could "catch" cancer from her. They outlined the types of precautions that would be necessary, and explained that Hannah would only be able to be there a couple of hours a day. She wouldn't be able to be in the regular classroom or in large group situations such as the cafeteria.

Her tutor would be providing instruction for her, and she would be set up in the guidance office, where other students would be able to join her for specific lessons as long as they were not actively ill, did careful hand-washing, and all equipment was disinfected. Her ability to fight infection was steadily increasing, as her ANC had risen to 900. She also had a platelet count of 140,000 which meant she was less at risk for bleeding. We did have to obtain special permission for an exception to the rule about no hats or caps in the classroom. Disey had been correct: Hannah had no real interest in wearing her wig to school, but continued to wear hats and scarves.

For the remainder of the fall semester, she attended school for two hours a day. Her tutor conducted her classes along with whoever could join her. Despite being out of school for the more than half the fall semester, Hannah was ahead of where the class was. She had become used to completing most of the week's assignments in a day or two while she was in the hospital, and spreading it out over the whole week was boring for her.

I was glad she felt well enough to be in school at all. Her reintegration socially was more important to me at this point than any class assignment. She had been isolated for a long time, her only new friendships being those she had developed over the last seven months with children who were ill with long-term illnesses and disabilities. It was important to resume a life among her peers and begin to move beyond the hospitalization experience.

I don't remember much about Thanksgiving, but I'm sure we ate something that resembled the great American feast. Unfortunately, Hannah had once again developed thrush and couldn't enjoy eating. We were also all still adjusting to living in the same house again. It was hard to believe we wouldn't be suddenly called back to the hospital. Hannah continued to need constant blood checks with frequent visits to MCCP in Scarborough, but that was easy compared to living on the inpatient unit. I still worried constantly, but at least I did so while resuming my life at home.

Each blood draw was torture. I spent the two or three days before each blood test worrying about what they would find and then walking around with a lump of molten lead in my stomach, holding my breath until we received the results telling us she didn't have any blast cells. In fact, I spent most of Thanksgiving Day quietly obsessing about the blood draw scheduled for the day after. Fortunately, the frequency of the blood checks was slowly being extended from every few days to once a week.

Hannah tired easily, and each time she was over-tired or said she didn't feel good, I became anxious. I quizzed her about exactly *how* she felt bad, and checked her for a fever while watching her closely until she seemed to feel better. Honestly, I hovered, became a "helicopter mom." It was hard not to be obsessive about something going wrong. Even though I wanted to be home, the worry was constant. I doubted myself and wondered if we would pay for my insistence that she be at home instead of in the hospital. Thankfully, as the time between checks was extended, Hannah had more good days than bad, and I became less obsessive.

By Christmas, we had been out of the hospital for more than a month. On some clinic visits, we had stopped by the hospital to say hello to staff. They were happy to see us and happy that Hannah wasn't there any more. She was looking less and less like a cancer patient. I had given her a buzz cut to even the length of her hair, and while some patches were black and curly, the newer hair was lighter and straight. With it all the same length, the two textures and colors weren't so obvious.

We felt like disaster survivors. We tended to huddle together touching each other for reassurance, happy to be alive and intact. I cried much more easily and became maudlin over Christmas ornaments, the sentiments on holiday cards, and TV commercials about families being together. Hannah and Caitlin laughed and teased each other as they began to reestablish their at-home relationship. Mike tended to tear up any time we talked about what had happened. Even though we had visitors, we were a pretty closed unit.

With the exception of Hannah's 12th birthday celebration, we weren't entertaining. Only family and close friends were there and there was an underlying sadness as thoughts of what might have been affected us all. We laughed louder than we should have and hid tears behind the whipped cream on our slices of strawberry-covered angel food cake. We caught each other stealing covert glances at Hannah just to reassure ourselves that she really was there and okay.

Hannah laughed with everyone, exclaimed over her presents, and graciously took the teasing about almost being a teenager, but she looked out at us from old, wise eyes which were still rimmed with the dark circles of illness. She had been a little girl at last year's birthday celebration, but was now an adult, if not by chronology, then by experience. Her childhood was a memory, its innocence lost forever.

Time was the best healer. Our lives slowly returned to normal as Hannah went back to her regular classroom in school. She had easily kept up with all of the classroom work, including science experiments such as dissecting a sheep's eyeball. She still couldn't be in the cafeteria, but otherwise had been reintegrated into middle-school life. As she became more confident about fitting in with her classmates, she relaxed about her hair and finally went to school one day in late spring without a hat or wig.

We had one more challenge as our daily fears about her survival began to lessen a bit: maintaining insurance coverage. True to Mike's concerns about working for a high-tech start-up, it became clear in late winter that there was a problem with the future of the company. They were initially scheduled to be bought out, but instead they essentially ceased to exist. This meant that until Mike was able to find another job, we would have to buy health insurance through COBRA. We spoke with many insurance carriers in the area and not one of them would agree to take Hannah on our family plan, citing a preexisting condition. I was grateful we still had coverage through the Katie Beckett program. Each carrier did assure us that this was considered credible coverage, and as long as there was no break in coverage, she would be eligible for an employer's group plan.

Privately, I ranted and raved again about the broken nature of our health care payment system. We had received the final bills from the hospital: counting everything that had been covered, the cost was around a million dollars. Without insurance coverage and the Katie Beckett funds as backup, we would be bankrupt. However, we were not yet in the clear. If Hannah relapsed before Mike found a job with insurance coverage, we could still face financial ruin. So it was a big relief when he found a new job that midsummer with a company that offered health insurance benefits. As soon as we had that, the Katie Beckett Funds stopped since she was no longer in active treatment. Now, for this and every other reason, we could only pray that she stayed in remission.

Chapter 22
REMEMBRANCE OF THINGS PAST

As the one-year anniversary of Hannah's diagnosis came closer, I found myself reliving all of the stages of finding out what was wrong with her. When I looked at pre-diagnosis pictures and recent ones, they could have been two different people. The child I saw before me now was tough and resilient, but had an underlying vulnerability. She had come close to death, but for now survived.

The months in the hospital had changed who she was, but in many ways she hadn't changed at all. Her sense of humor and quick wit had survived and in fact sharpened. She looked after her own needs and kept her own counsel. She was still a voracious reader and loved to discuss new ideas, and she channeled some of this into a debate society, which she started with the friends who ate lunch in the classroom with her every day. She had strong opinions and no qualms about voicing them.

Even though she was regaining some sense of control over her world, it was still a struggle to leave the last months behind. She never saw herself as a victim of cancer, and refused to define herself as a survivor. She coped with cancer and the treatment by seeing it as some terrible parallel world full of medical problems and unpleasant experiences. When it was over, she went back to being a person again. It seemed a sensible coping mechanism.

At this one year milestone, she had a complete medical check-up, which included a cardiology workup. There were no blast cells in her blood and no evidence of heart damage from the Danorubicin. I wanted to celebrate, but was afraid to. Instead, I felt like walking around with my fingers, toes, and eyes crossed in hopes of warding off bad luck.

Hannah's energy level wasn't always high, but she continued to grow stronger. It was, at times, hard to fathom that just a year ago she had been fighting for her life and we couldn't believe this time would ever come. Mike and I still worried constantly and kept her very close, but we were starting to relax as the summer progressed.

In mid-June, she received an invitation to attend the Hole in the Wall Gang Camp in Ashford, Connecticut. We knew little about it, only that it was started by Paul Newman to provide children with cancer and other diseases such as hemophilia and sickle cell disease a summer camp experience. We looked it up on the Internet and took the virtual tour. It looked fantastic. There were expert medical staff and an almost one-to-one staff-to-camper ratio. With her recent history, we had not imagined Hannah being able to attend *any* camp.

Deciding we would risk letting her attend camp was probably the most therapeutic thing we did for all of us. However, for me, accepting the need to do it and being willing to let her go were two different things. I felt we had kept her alive by sheer force of will, and if we didn't maintain a constant, high-level, intense effort, she still might die. I feared any lack of vigilance would result in relapse. Frankly, the thought of letting someone else care for her without my being there really scared me.

Hannah was very excited about going and had finished packing by the Wednesday before the Saturday start of camp. Having been in control of so much of her life over the last year, I tried to help, but she deftly pointed out that she had the camp list of what to bring and had it all organized. I knew she was capable, but I had trouble not micromanaging her life. Perhaps it wasn't surprising that she was ready to move on before I was, but I was emotionally unprepared for the suddenness of the change.

The trip to camp took around three hours, and once we crossed the border from Massachusetts into Connecticut and exited the interstate, we were driving through picturesque old New England villages and past small farms. It was beautiful, and some of my qualms about Hannah going to camp lessened. If the camp was like this, I could imagine it being a healing environment.

As we crested a hill, we saw the Hole in the Wall Gang sign, and people dressed in Hawaiian garb, holding balloons and signs. Mike braked sharply to make the turn into the camp road. He put down his window as they all came running over to the car laughing and shouting.

"Which one is our camper?" asked a girl dressed in a grass skirt.

We all pointed at Hannah.

"First time?"

Hannah nodded without saying anything.

"Welcome! Welcome! Welcome! You're going to love it!"

Hannah shrank back into her seat. She looked out her window, not making eye contact with any of us. My doubts returned.

I took a deep breath and, as had been my habit during Hannah's treatment, when anxious, I switched into cheerful-upbeat mode.

"Well at least it looks like they expect to have a great week."

Hannah gave me a sour look and didn't respond.

We waited in the line of cars stopping to receive information and directions to parking. We slowly inched forward into the area in front of the registration building. A counselor bounded over to the car and motioned Mike to stop. Concerned about holding up the line, Mike signaled asking if we should really stop here and the young man nodded an emphatic yes.

Mike had barely put the car into Park when the young man pulled open the car door shouting, "Which one is our new camper?"

Caitlin pointed at Hannah, who hesitantly smiled and nodded.

"What's your name?" he asked.

"Uh, Hannah Glover."

He quickly checked his clipboard list. "You're in Purple! That's a great group of cabins! You'll love being in Purple! Come on out and let's get your bags."

"Shouldn't we park the car first?" Mike asked.

"Nope. Just unload here."

Caitlin and I got out with Hannah while Mike popped the trunk so that we could get the bags.

The young greeter accompanied Hannah to the registration table and introduced her to a counselor sporting a purple lanyard.

"You're in Purple! I'm a counselor in Purple! Step over here and get your ID picture taken. You're gonna love Purple!"

Hannah complied, but clearly had some doubts about all this enthusiasm. She and Caitlin were nearly joined at the hip as we waited for a ride to the center of camp. Her luggage was loaded into a brightly decorated covered wagon near the horse stables for its own journey.

After a review of medications and medical needs, we were ready to head to the infirmary for a checkup with the medical staff. As I watched the procession of campers checking in, I began to choke up. Having lived around children with cancer over the last year, there was no mistaking the nature of the illnesses these children had been through. I watched Hannah looking at other kids who looked like her. Many were wearing bandanas or hats over bald heads, and if they did have hair, it was short and new or patchy and sparse.

As we stood there, we heard snatches of discussions about central lines and equipment needed for the week. I was saved from embarrassing Hannah with open weeping by Mike's arrival from the car park. He put his arm around me and gave a quick hug as an electric golf cart arrived. A cheerful counselor bid us climb aboard, and we traveled downhill away from the stables and registration area onto a wide, gravel road which wound through beautiful old shade trees.

The driver pointed to a road that disappeared through the trees in the direction of the lake and said, "That's where Mr. Newman lives when he's here."

I whispered in Caitlin's ear, "Mr. Newman? Who's Mr. Newman?"

She gave me an astounded look, "*Paul* Newman, Mom. I can't believe you don't know that."

I laughed at myself and said, "Oh, *that* Mr. Newman. I don't think I've ever heard him referred to as anything but *Paul* Newman."

As we rode on, Hannah, Caitlin, and I talked about one of their favorite movies, *Butch Cassidy and the Sundance Kid,* and how the Hole in the Wall Gang was the name of their hideout. As we arrived in the camp proper, we saw buildings ahead of us that looked as if they had come directly from the set of the movie. I didn't know if Hannah was excited about being there yet, but I definitely felt this would be a great week for her.

After she had been checked over by the health staff, a staff person came to walk us to the Purple group cabins. She had been a volunteer here before, and reassured us that the kids had a great time, were well cared for, and would want to return again and again.

We entered a clearing with three carbon-copy log cabins facing each other. All of the doors and trim on the cabins were purple, but the rail porches were natural wood. Inside, the large sitting area had comfortable couches and chairs, and the walls were lined with shelves containing crafts and books.

The large, rectangular bunk room to the right of the main room had beds along each wall with four sets of bunk beds in the corners and two single beds across from each other along the side walls. There was also a rocking chair under the large window at the end of the room. A couple of beds had already been claimed, but both the single beds were free. Hannah decided on one of these. Each bed had a trunk at the end for storing personal items, and on top of each trunk was a beautiful handmade quilt or afghan which was a gift to the camper. There was also a "goodie" bag with water bottle, stuffed animal, snacks, a journal, and some toiletry articles.

At the suggestion of the counselors, we went to the center of camp for lunch while Hannah settled in. When we returned, she was already involved in a craft project and chatting with two of her cabin mates. She was fine. The counselor said they would send us a postcard during the week, reminding us not to call unless it was absolutely necessary. If we did need to check on her, one of them would call us back. After lots of hugs and kisses and for me, quickly swallowed tears, we left.

We declined a ride to the parking lot, preferring to walk and stretch our legs a bit before getting back into the car. Other families were still arriving as we left, but it was a trickle rather than the previous torrent. Our drive home was somber, but we talked about all of the fun we could imagine Hannah having. Unfortunately, thoughts about what brought her here and what we were doing last year at this time still cast a shadow over everything. The long months since Hannah was diagnosed still felt unreal. It was hard to allow ourselves to think about much of what had happened when she was in treatment, and the full impact hadn't hit us even now.

This week, while Hannah was away, Caitlin would be the center of our attention. She had sacrificed a lot in this process, and now I was looking forward to being with her. I hoped that for a brief time my children could just be children again. Since Caitlin had swim practice, we dropped her off in Dover and then Mike and I drove home alone to an empty house.

It had been fourteen months since we'd both been away from Hannah at the same time. From the day of her diagnosis a year ago, with the exception of the few hours each day in school this spring and our one night at the Ronald McDonald House, one of us had been physically with her either in the hospital or at home. Sitting on the floor together in the living room, we talked about the enormity of what we had accomplished.

All the unshed tears of the last year couldn't be held back any more. We hugged each other and sobbed. We had cried many times during treatment, but had never dared to really admit how angry, scared, and depressed we were for fear we wouldn't be able to keep going. For the first time since receiving that awful phone call, I didn't need to be in control. Crying finally provided an inner release and I grieved.

AFTERWORD
Fall 2010

Cancer no longer dominates our daily lives and we are stronger as a result of the lessons given us. We recognize the importance of living life fully, taking joy in what really matters, and saying "I love you" as often as we can to those who matter most. Our memories continue to fade from present to past, losing much of their terror with the passage of time.

Each of us is changed in different ways as a result of Hannah's treatment. We may harbor fears about the future, but have learned to live in the present by reminding ourselves of how lucky we were. By talking about the good things that happened, we were able to blunt the pain. We escaped the fate of over 50% of families who have a child in cancer treatment: Mike and I are still married and our romance lives on.

Hannah is in her second year of college after graduating high school as valedictorian of her class. She is focusing on the sciences, but thinks she may want to teach or work in public health. She is a talented writer, and who knows if she may one day write her own book on childhood cancer treatment.

The Hole in the Wall gang camp was full the second summer after her treatment ended. They offered her an alternate camp experience with the Ocean Classrooms Foundation learning to sail aboard the schooner, *Harvey Gamage*. Twice more she found ways to sail with them, having fallen in love with large wooden sailing ships. While she hasn't yet decided what she will do in life, sailing will be part of the equation.

She never saw herself as a victim of cancer. It was simply a part of her childhood, and she didn't feel sorry for herself or want to make it important. She has continued to be a remarkable, resilient human being.

Caitlin graduated college with honors in chemistry. She did volunteer teaching in China after college and says the most important thing to her is using her life to make a difference in the world. She is currently doing research in water remediation for the developing world in a Ph.D.

program in civil engineering.

She always believed Hannah wouldn't die, because there wasn't any way we would let that happen. Her positive belief in a good outcome, along with her love and support, were, I believe, a significant part of Hannah's healing.

Mike continues to commute to Massachusetts, and the journey has been improved by being able to ride the train to Boston where he develops cell phone applications for Google. He gave up soccer after a severe injury during a game but continues to run daily, and his new love is the 200-mile team relay "Reach the Beach" race.

He feels we were lucky in Hannah's survival, and although he would never have chosen to have this experience, it gave him many gifts. One of the most important was the opportunity to be together as father and daughter, sharing books, movies, and stories during the long hours spent in the hospital. He says he doesn't like to think about the good times before Hannah was diagnosed, because if we were back there, we would have to go through the trauma again.

Once Mike and I knew what was involved in her treatment and care, we saw it as a task to be accomplished and set about doing it with a vengeance. We recognized that being her advocate and never leaving her to face the challenges of treatment alone were two of the most important things we could do. I believe the nursing care I provided her while she was in treatment and immediately after contributed to a positive outcome, but more importantly, it gave me a way to cope.

We were reminded of how close we came to losing Hannah when a boy from our community died of AML. He was diagnosed post-mortem and didn't have a chance to be treated. He too was an athlete, and although he had bruising and several other symptoms, it wasn't what anyone was looking for. We were distressed by the news, and as we stood with his family at the funeral home, it brought back our fear. Had I not insisted on the blood work and testing, would we still be grieving Hannah's death?

It has made me want to tell every parent that a fatigued child with bruising or petechiae (pinpoint-sized red spots under the skin), headaches, loss of appetite, or frequent infections needs to be medically evaluated. A complete blood count is not an expensive test. Early treatment *does* make a difference. There will be about 43,050 new cases of leukemia diagnosed in the United States this year; 5300 of those cases will be in children. While the most common childhood leukemia is ALL, 20% is caused by AML. The incidence of cancer is, unfortunately, rising, and an easy solution to the problem is not readily at hand. The good news is that the survival rate has improved and new research continues to hold hope for better treatment options. When I hear the current debate on genetics and stem-cell research, I am irked by the willingness to indulge in demagoguery and ideology instead of considering the consequences to people, especially children like Hannah.

After spending time teaching nursing at the university and writing, I have returned to private family practice and enjoy the opportunity to treat and care for others. Having so poignantly experienced the other side of the system has altered my practice as a Nurse Practitioner. While I had always been caring and concerned about the needs of the patients I treated, I have a new sensitivity to what it feels like to be on the powerless side of the bed.

Giving a diagnosis to anyone should be a well-thought-out process humanized by expressions of empathy and understanding. I try to remember how I wanted to be treated when we were facing Hannah's diagnosis, and while it may cost me some of my leisure hours completing the paperwork later, I spend extra time with anyone coping with a frightening medical situation. I haven't had to give anyone a diagnosis of cancer, but I have worked with patients who have been recently diagnosed and I can genuinely feel what they are experiencing.

When I contribute something to the care of others, it is as if I am repaying some of the huge debt for the kindness and care we received. The lesson of *how* to receive, and not just to give, still eludes me. I did, however, learn an important lesson about the ways in which I can avoid putting others in my debt when I provide their care. I let them know that it is a two-way street and that I am given much by being able to use my skills as a healer. I thank them for enriching my life by being who they are.

When Hannah's treatment finished, we had many reasons to be happy. She had survived with no long-term disabilities. We remained an intact family and hadn't lost everything to the cost of treatment. Still, it took a long time to recover emotionally. My trust in the universe and the fairness of life was badly shaken and in opposition to how I had previously viewed the world: the glass is now half empty.

My knowledge of grief and grieving theory was just words compared to living it. We remained isolated, and while the emotional scars weren't visible, they were there. I discovered through the process of writing this book that memoir writing provided a mechanism for awakening order from emotional chaos. Each subsequent draft arrayed the fractured pieces into a framework through which the work of grieving could begin to heal my soul.

Love is a rigorous master. When I chose to have children, I chose to give my heart into the care of others. The opportunity to love my children has given me astounding joy and unnamed gifts of richness and meaning beyond compare. If Hannah had not been diagnosed with cancer, I wouldn't have understood the depth of that love and the terror the fear of losing a child lodged in my heart. As long as she continues to survive and grow into the wonderful young woman she is becoming, I will gratefully live with that fear for the rest of my life.

Although Hannah has remained in remission since that first round of chemotherapy, we continue to be skeptically optimistic. As we celebrate the eighth year since diagnosis, we are starting to believe it turned out okay. We continue to live one day at a time, giving back for our good fortune whenever and wherever we can, while remembering John Lennon's words: "Life is what happens while you're making plans."

ACKNOWLEDGEMENTS

It is with deep gratitude that we thank all of those who so generously helped us during Hannah's illness. We are blessed to live in a community of givers. Hannah received healing energy from prayer circles throughout this country and a Tibetan prayer wheel. We owe a debt of gratitude to all of the A negative platelet and blood donors, who literally gave of themselves. The Oyster River and Berwick Academy school communities, the swim and soccer team communities and all those on the help list made it possible for us to focus on caring for Hannah. To our families and friends scattered across the country, and Hannah and Caitlin's surrogate grandparents, Ken and Florence Potito and their extended family, your love and support sustained us.